Food, Health and Identity

D1578699

By addressing the issue of what we eat today, *Food, Health and Identity* considers the way in which our food habits are changing, and shows how our social and personal identities and our perception of health and risk influence our choices.

The Introduction seeks to indicate how social scientists can help us understand why people eat what they do. The following chapters, written by well-known anthropologists and sociologists, discuss themes of change and continuity in food and eating – the family meal, wedding cakes, nostalgia and the invention of tradition, the 'creolisation' of British food, and increases in vegetarianism and eating out. A second theme is that of identity, with studies of both ethnic minorities and the dominant majority, as well as the creation of individual identity through culinary lifestyle. Finally, questions of health and risk perception are addressed in discussions of current 'healthy eating' advice and the way in which people respond to it, including a study of recent BSE crises in the context of government/media relations and the new environmental radicalism.

Food, Health and Identity is based on recent field research. It addresses topical issues which are central to the study of anthropology, sociology and health promotion.

Pat Caplan is Professor of Social Anthropology at Goldsmiths' College, University of London.

Food, Health and Identity

Edited by Pat Caplan

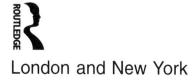

London and New York

First published 1997 by Routledge
11 New Fetter Lane, London EC4P 4EE

Simultaneously published in the USA and Canada
by Routledge
29 West 35th Street, New York, NY 10001

Typeset in Times by Keystroke, Jacaranda Lodge, Wolverhampton
Printed and bound in Great Britain by Biddles Ltd, Guildford and
King's Lynn

British Library Cataloguing in Publication Data
A catalogue record for this book is available from the British Library

Library of Congress Cataloging in Publication Data
Food, health, and identity / edited by Pat Caplan.
      p.   cm.
   Includes bibliographical references and index.
   1. Food habits—Great Britain. 2. Diet—Great Britain.
I. Caplan, Patricia.
GT2853.G7F66 1997
394.1′2′0941—dc21   96–51909
                                              CIP

ISBN 0–415–15679–3 (hbk)
ISBN 0–415–15680–7 (pbk)

Contents

Contributors

Hannah Bradby is a researcher at the MRC Medical Sociology Unit at Glasgow University where her main areas of interest are ethnicity, and religion and health, particularly in young people.

Pat Caplan is Professor of Anthropology at Goldsmiths' College, London. She has carried out fieldwork in Tanzania and South Asia and her recent books include *Gendered Fields* (with D. Bell and W.J. Karim; Routledge 1994), *Understanding Disputes* (Berg 1995), and *African Voices, African Lives* (Routledge 1997). She has had a long-standing interest in the anthropology of food and published *Feasts, Fasts and Famines* (Berg 1995). From 1992 to 1996, she directed the two 'Concepts of Healthy Eating' projects, funded by the ESRC, which involved comparative studies carried out in South-East London and West Wales.

Simon Charsley is a social anthropologist in the Department of Sociology at Glasgow University. His fieldwork-based research has been in Uganda, Scotland and India. He is the author of *The Princes of Nyakysua* (East Africa Publishing House 1969), *Culture and Sericulture* (Academic Press 1982), *Rites of Marrying* (Manchester University Press 1991), *Wedding Cakes and Cultural History* (Routledge 1992), and articles on these and other topics. He is currently concerned chiefly with the study of development amongst former 'Untouchables' in southern India.

Simon Cohn came to Goldsmiths' College to work on a research project on patient perceptions of health care in the UK National Health Service. His own PhD research looked at concepts of health and disease amongst people with diabetes. His current interests include medical anthropology, individualism in western society, and visual anthropology and representation. He has been centrally involved with the applied anthropology group, Anthropology in Action.

Nick Fiddes did his doctorate in the Department of Anthropology at the University of Edinburgh, where he is currently an Honorary Research Fellow. He is the author of *Meat: A Natural Symbol* (Routledge 1991) and has recently completed ESRC-funded ethnographic research into the culture of the new ecological protest movement in the UK.

Lynn Harbottle is a medical anthropologist and nutritionist. She worked in Papua New Guinea prior to employment in the NHS and later at Sheffield University, where she undertook a dietary survey of British Pakistani and Bangladeshi weanlings. Her current research explores the use of food as a marker of ethnicity and its role in gendered power relations through the work of Iranian migrants. Recent articles include 'Feminism and medical anthropology' (1995), '"Palship", parties and pilgrimage: kinship, community formation and self-transformation of Iranian migrants to Britain' (1995) and 'Towards a culturally sensitive research approach' (1996).

Allison James is a Senior Lecturer in Applied Anthropology at the University of Hull. She has published a number of articles on the anthropology of food and her other main research area is in childhood studies. She is author of *Childhood Identities* (Edinburgh University Press 1993) and joint author of *Growing Up and Growing Old* (Sage 1993).

Anne Keane was a Research Associate in the Anthropology Department, Goldsmiths' College from 1992 to 1995, working on the 'Concepts of Healthy Eating' project, part of the ESRC research programme 'The Nation's Diet: The Social Science of Food Choice'. She is currently completing her PhD thesis on food and the body.

Lydia Martens is lecturer in the Department of Applied Social Studies at the University of Paisley. Between 1994 and 1996 she worked as Research Associate in the Department of Sociology, Lancaster University.

David Miller is a member of the Stirling Media Research Institute. He is the author of *Don't Mention the War: Northern Ireland,*

Propaganda and the Media (Pluto 1994), editor (with Bill Rolston) of *War and Words: The Northern Ireland Media Reader* (Belfast: Beyond the Pale Publications 1996) and author (with the Glasgow Media Group) of *Dying of Ignorance: AIDS, the Media and Public Belief* (forthcoming).

Anne Murcott has an MA in social anthropology and a PhD in sociology. Her most recent book is *The Sociology of Food: Diet, Eating and Culture* (with Stephen Mennell and Anneke van Otterloo, Sage 1992) and she edited the international journal *Sociology of Health & Illness* from 1982–87. Currently she is Director of the ESRC (UK) research programme 'The Nation's Diet: The Social Science of Food Choice' and holds a research post as Professor of the Sociology of Health at South Bank University, London.

Jacquie Reilly is a researcher in the Department of Sociology at Glasgow University. Her research interests have centred on the production, content and reception of media messages in particular on food safety issues. Current research includes a project on the ESRC Risk Initiative entitled 'The Media and Expert Constructions of Risk' which is investigating the processes leading to the formation of accounts of risks and how these impact on public policy. Main publications include 'Food "scares" in the media' (Glasgow University Media Group 1994), 'Making an issue of food safety: the media, pressure groups and the public sphere' (in Donna Maura and Jeffrey Sobal (eds) *Food Eating and Nutrition as Social Problems: Constructivist Perspectives*, New York: Aldine De Gruyter 1995).

Alan Warde is Professor of Sociology at the University of Lancaster. He recently completed the project 'Eating Out and Eating In' under the ESRC's research programme 'The Nation's Diet: The Social Science of Food Choice'. Research on food stems from an interest in the sociology of consumption on which he has written a number of articles. His new book, *Consumption, Food and Taste: Culinary Antinomies and Commodity Culture*, will be published by Sage in the spring of 1997.

Anna Willetts was a Research Associate in the Anthropology Department, Goldsmiths' College, from 1992 to 1995, working on the 'Concepts of Healthy Eating' project, part of the ESRC research programme 'The Nation's Diet: The Social Science of

Food Choice'. She is currently working as a researcher on food for a national consumer organisation and is writing her PhD thesis.

Janice Williams did her doctorate at the University of Sussex, studying orthodox Jews in Britain and Israel, and published her thesis under the title *Conceptual Change and Religious Practice* (Avebury 1987). She has worked in television and the health service. From 1994 to 1996, she was a Research Associate at Goldsmiths' College on the 'Concepts of Healthy Eating' Project, Phase II, carrying out fieldwork in her native Wales. She is currently working on her family's farm and continuing to write up her data, as well as teaching part-time at the University of Swansea.

Preface and acknowledgements

A book such as this, written by anthropologists and sociologists with first-hand experience of carrying out field-work on food practices in the British context today, would have been difficult to compile until recently. Although anthropology has a long interest in the study of food, it has relatively rarely been one in food *per se*. Following Lévi-Strauss's dictum that food is 'good to think with', it has rather been seen as a way of understanding social and cultural processes. Furthermore, anthropology has mainly focused its attentions on 'other', mainly non-western societies, and only recently, with a few honourable exceptions, have ethnographers begun to carry out anthropology 'at home'. Thus paradoxically, at the time of writing, it would be possible to compile a much more detailed account of the anthropology of food in, say, India, than it is of food in Britain.

It was for this reason that when, in 1995, I was invited to convene a day-long panel on a subject of my own choosing at the British Association for the Advancement of Science annual conference, I selected the topic of 'Food in Britain' from a social science viewpoint. Several of the contributors to that panel were carrying out research for a project entitled 'Concepts of Healthy Eating' (Caplan, Keane, Willetts and Williams), while Murcott was the Director of the ESRC Research Progamme of which that project was a part ('The Nation's Diet: The Social Science of Food Choice'). Other contributors had already carried on research and published on food in Britain as had Murcott herself. All of their BAAS papers are included in this collection. In addition, several new contributors joined the book project: Martens and Warde, and Reilly were also carrying out research for their own projects as part of 'The Nation's Diet' programme, while three young researchers (Bradby, Cohn and Harbottle) were studying food practices as part of their doctoral research.

I am grateful to the contributors for all their efforts and thank them for their patience. Thanks are also due to the ESRC, which has not only funded many of the research projects represented in this collection, but also gave some funding for the original BAAS panel. Karen Catling, the project secretary on the 'Concepts of Healthy Eating' projects, played a major role in the organisation of the BAAS panel, and has also assisted in the production of this book in numerous other ways. Susan Greenwood assisted with the converting of different word processing packages into a common format. I am also grateful to the editorial team at Routledge, Heather Gibson, Fiona Bailey and Eleanor Jackson, with whom it has been a pleasure to work.

Pat Caplan
September 1996

Chapter 1

Approaches to the study of food, health and identity

Pat Caplan

In this introduction, I seek to suggest ways in which social scientists can begin to make sense of the bewildering variety of eating practices discernible in one western society today – Britain. The chapter begins by outlining how anthropologists have approached this topic, looking particularly at the legacy of the structuralists as well as their critics who adopt a more historical and materialist approach, and then turning to some more recent post-structuralist approaches. It next examines three themes which arise out of the papers in this volume: changing food practices and their implications, food as a marker of identity and difference, and the relationship between food and health. The discussion also includes issues which have recently become significant such as risk and lifestyle. The chapter argues that the study of food reveals our social and cultural selves, as well as our individual subjectivities.

FOOD AS LANGUAGE, FOOD AS SYSTEM

Anthropologists began to write a good deal about food with the rise of structuralism in the 1960s,[1] particularly following the work of Lévi-Strauss (1965, 1968, 1970). He and his followers sought to understand food as a cultural system, an approach which clearly recognises that 'taste' is culturally shaped and socially controlled. There is by now a considerable literature influenced by his structuralist approach which treats food as analogous to language, and examines the ways in which its meanings can be grasped from an understanding of symbol and metaphor. Lévi-Strauss maintained that food was 'good to think with' and that deciphering the codes underlying such matters as food enabled the anthropologist to reach 'a significant knowledge of the unconscious attitudes of the society or societies under consideration' (1968: 87). This kind of work has produced important insights into the rules underlying everyday life, perhaps most famously in Lévi-Strauss's own work on the raw and the cooked (1970).

Roland Barthes also utilised a linguistic analogy in the understanding of food, searching for a code or 'grammar'. Barthes sees food as a sign as well as a need and indeed the need itself is highly structured: 'Substances, techniques of preparation, habits, all become part of a system of differences in signification; and as soon as this happens, we have communication by way of food' (1975: 51). Indeed, he suggests that an entire 'world' (social environment) is present in and signified by food. His basic argument in this context, as in others, is that where there is meaning, there must be system, an argument to which we will be returning later.

Mary Douglas was influenced by both Lévi-Strauss and Barthes, but developed their work in slightly different directions. She has published on food throughout her career, beginning with an analysis of the Jewish dietary prohibitions laid down in the book of Leviticus (1966). Drawing upon anthropological work on classification, Douglas sought to show that animals such as pigs were forbidden to the Hebrews because they were creatures considered to be anomalous under a system of classification based upon chewing the cud and cloven-footedness, and therefore impure or polluting.

In some of her subsequent work Douglas has focused on British food and on the constitution of a meal (Douglas and Nicod 1974, Douglas 1975). She argues that one will discover the social boundaries which food meanings encode according to their position in a series such as a single day (breakfast through to nightcap), a week (encompassing the Sunday dinner), an annual series (which includes holidays and fast days), and a life-cycle series (from christening to funeral). Douglas explains that meals are ordered in scale or importance and grandeur through the day, the week and the year, but the smallest, meanest meal metonymically figures the structure of the grandest (1975). Such an analysis, then, illuminates cultural views not only on what constitutes food, but how we eat it. She argues that food and eating are symbolic of a particular social order, thus the patterns she discusses stand for much more than themselves.

The anthropological work on food published during the 1960s and 1970s remains important and influential; it shows clearly that culture plays a significant role in determining what we classify as food. However, such work does not tell us everything we might want to know. For example, it does little to explain the social relationships of power which are involved in food transactions, or changes in food habits, as several writers began to point out in the 1980s (Goody 1982, Mennell 1985, Mintz 1985).

In his work, *Cooking, Cuisine and Class* (1982), Jack Goody criticises a Lévi-Straussian approach for its emphasis on culture, and for failing to consider social relations and individual differences; he also takes issue with Douglas for neglecting internal social differentiation, as well as external socio-cultural influences, historical factors and material elements. Goody acknowledges the importance of culture, but he argues that a study of food and eating must involve political economy both at the micro-level, such as the household, through to the macro-level, such as states and their formation and structure.

Sidney Mintz has an approach which is in many ways rather similar to that of Goody. Taking a single food item – sugar – he considers changes in eating habits in the West over the past several hundred years, focusing particularly on the nineteenth and twentieth centuries, during which period the amount of sugar consumed has increased dramatically. For Mintz, sugar is a metaphor for social relations, for instance between the producers of sugar, the owners of plantations originally built upon African slavery, and consumers of the commodity in the West. Like Goody, he does not ignore the cultural dimension, but he makes history central to his analysis.

While some of the anthropological literature of the 1970s may be criticised for ignoring both historical change and social relations, including those of politics and economics, it remains extremely influential as, for example, Fürst *et al.*'s 1991 collection on food in northern Europe indicates. Although today most anthropologists have taken on board the need to situate their work in the context of historical changes and political economy, there is still a search for meaning, which can be reached through the use of metaphor, metonymy and symbol, as we will find in the articles in this book. In other words, food is never 'just food' and its significance can never be purely nutritional. Furthermore, it is intimately bound up with social relations, including those of power, of inclusion and exclusion, as well as with cultural ideas about classification (including food and non-food, the edible and the inedible), the human body and the meaning of health.

CHANGING FOOD PRACTICES

Changes in consumption[2] and their effects, particularly on health, have been an important theme in much recent writing on food. One debate concerns the extent to which palatability coincides not only with edibility, but also with desirability from a nutritional viewpoint. Some nutritionists, such as Yudkin and McKenzie (1964), have maintained that humans like to eat what is good for them. More recently, some anthropologists, notably Marvin Harris and Eric Ross, have also argued that humans tend to choose what is good for them nutritionally on the grounds of evolutionary selectivity and adaptation (Harris 1985, Harris and Ross 1987). Others have demonstrated that such a link is tenuous and argued for the importance of culture as a determining factor in taste. They point to the huge range of potentially edible items which are ignored in every culture. Leach (1964), for instance, notes that Westerners do not eat animals which are either far away and out of our control, nor animals which are very close because they are 'like us'; indeed, the British treat certain animals, such as dogs and horses, as taboo. Sahlins, too, notes that 'edibility is inversely related to humanity' (1976: 175). This explains the strength of the taboo on eating cat or dog meat, which is also discussed by Goody in the light of his own experience as a prisoner of war (1982: 83–5).

Mintz has also argued that human beings have, by and large, eaten what is good for them until relatively recently in human history (1992, 1994). He notes that there are three basic types of food which have been around for a long time all over the world. These are the complex carbohydrates such as rice, wheat, potatoes, yams, taro, sorghum; second, the flavour-giving foods which help the carbohydrate go down; third, protein-carrying plants such as peas, beans and pulses. These he refers to as *core, fringe* and *legume* (CFL) and he argues that they form a basic pattern in all human food. But, he notes, the basic CFL pattern began to crumble in western Europe during the time of the Industrial Revolution and the pattern has decayed more rapidly since that time over greater areas of the world. The major reason why this has happened is that an increasing amount of two alternative foods have entered our diets in the form of fat, of both animal and plant origin, and sugar:

> Fats and sugar – both in the way that they are extracted, and in the ways that they are conceived and combined – have modified

in some ways our human relationship to nature, while playing a special role in the remaking of the food habits of the entire world.

(1992: 18)

In his earlier work, *Sweetness and Power* (1985), Mintz showed that the increased consumption of sugar during the nineteenth and twentieth centuries detracted considerably from nutrition. This process has accelerated in the latter part of the twentieth century with the rise of food technology and the merging of the agricultural and chemical industries. In other words, palatability and nutrition have become quite distinct, summed up in the advertising slogan 'Naughty but nice'.

Furthermore, Mintz (1984, 1985) has also suggested that the great increase in the eating of already-prepared food inside and outside the home is having a profound effect on our lives. He notes that such forms of eating are touted as the ultimate in 'freedom of individual choice' but argues that in 'eating without meals', eating has been desocialised. As a result of this development, there is a move away from the kind of lexicon or grammar of food suggested in the work of anthropologists such as Mary Douglas, with the dissolving of the structure of the meal into a pattern of ragged and discontinous but frequent snacks, or what the food marketers have come to call 'grazing'. In this process, Mintz suggests, the entire productive character of societies is being recast, and with it, the 'very nature of time, of work, and of leisure' (1985: 213).

Mintz is thus pessimistic about the future of food and eating, not only in terms of health, but also in terms of the social relations which are fostered by commensality. For him modern food habits appear symptomatic of alienation. The French anthropologist Fischler has also spoken of 'gastro-anomie' in modern western food habits (1980).

But such conclusions may be premature: perhaps, as Barthes (1975) has suggested, we first need to look for patterns, and where we do we will find meaning. Such patterns may be infinitely more complex than those suggested by the early work on meals by Douglas, but it is unlikely that they do not exist, that people do not invest modern food with meaning, or that food has been totally divorced from social relationships.

In a recent study of the eating patterns of Canadian teenagers, for example, Chapman and Maclean (1993) find that they divide food into two categories: junk food and good food. The latter is associated with family meals and the domestic setting, the former with peer groups and fun. Thus even though teenagers are aware that junk food is not 'good for you' in a health sense – indeed they express concern about weight gain and skin problems which might flow from its consumption – nonetheless they do eat it because of what it represents: freedom from parental restraint and good times with their friends. Similarly, in her work on children's sweets, Allison James suggests that such items are treated by children as a means of resistance to adult norms (James 1982). Here again, then, food is like language – its meaning can shift according to contexts of time and place and people can switch food codes just as they do language codes, depending on with whom they are communicating at any point in time.

One change to which Mintz alludes and which is frequently discussed in the media is the end of the family meal, often associated with the demise of the family. Yet the evidence from recent studies of food in the West is that the meal remains an important template in most households (Murcott 1982, 1983, DeVault 1991, Charles and Kerr 1988). Young people who may have spent a large part of their teenage years living on snacks and fast food appear likely to change their habits when they move in with a partner, and particularly when they begin having children (Keane and Willetts 1995, Backett *et al.* 1994). Even in families where all members do not sit around a table every day, the meal retains its symbolic significance. Indeed, having a 'proper meal' may actually add to its importance once it becomes a less frequent occurrence. Several articles in this collection, notably those by Martens and Warde, Williams and James, note the symbolic importance of the meal, regardless of the frequency with which it is consumed.

In her article in this volume, Murcott addresses the frequent complaints about the demise of the meal in Britain, noting that there has long been a gap between rhetoric and reality: for example, upper-class children in the nineteenth and first part of the twentieth centuries ate quite separately from adults, first at home in the nursery, and then, if boys, at boarding school. She shows that concern about the supposedly declining institution of the family meal has been in evidence in both Britain and the USA since before the Second World War. Murcott thus suggests that the meal stands as a very powerful metaphor for 'the family', and its 'decline' must therefore be read as a 'standing item on the agenda of twentieth century public commentary on the nature of family life', a fact which counters Falk's recent contention that in complex societies, the meal is much less significant than in 'primitive' (sic) societies (1994).

Several other articles in this book also deal with issues of culinary change and continuity. Those by Martens and Warde, and by Williams, consider the great increase in eating outside of the home in recent years. But such changes also incorporate continuities: for example Williams finds that many people on holiday deliberately seek out food which is 'nostalgic', while Martens and Warde suggest that there are significant conceptual links between eating in a restaurant, and private notions of hospitality. James looks at the way in which British food has adopted certain kinds of 'foreign' items in recent years, leading to its apparent 'creolisation', but also argues that there are parallels with earlier adaptations and that the more recent ones have not changed its fundamental character. Bradby considers the extent to which young women of Punjabi origin living in Glasgow utilise not only an allopathic discourse around diet, but also make creative use of humoral models drawn from Ayurvedic and Unani systems; in this dynamic synthesis, there are both divergences from and continuities with the practices of their parents and grandparents.

Another recent change is considered by Fiddes and Willetts who both examine the large increase in vegetarianism in Britain, albeit from rather different viewpoints. Fiddes notes that concern for animals has always been a metaphor for other discourses and he sees a change in food habits as symbolising important shifts in society as a whole: 'these issues are suffused with layers of contemporary debate, which touch on much else besides the immediately apparent points at stake' (p. 259). Willetts, on the other hand, argues that many meat-eaters do share the same ethical concerns as *soi-disant* vegetarians, and that many of the latter, at least in her sample, actually eat meat from time to time. Her article raises not only the well-trodden theme in food research of the problematic relationship between beliefs and behaviour, but also that of lifestyle as identity, a topic discussed below.

Charsley, like Fiddes, is interested in the wider meanings of a particular food item, in his case the three-tier Victorian wedding cake which reached its apogee towards the end of the nineteenth century, and continued to be the classic form until quite recently. In his book *Wedding Cakes and Cultural History* (1992), Charsley noted that it was difficult to elicit meanings from informants who used such cakes at their own weddings. In his chapter here, however, he suggests that although the development of the cake related to a range of considerations and factors, 'key features were directly meaningful in relation to marriage ... because they were part of patterns of wider scope developing at the period' (p. 59). He argues that marriage in the nineteenth century was externally defined, especially for the middle classes – it was a 'heavily sanctioned common pattern' accurately symbolised by the essentially uniform cake. Yet this was not without its problems in a period where 'female passionlessness' was expected to be the norm, and there was a strong rhetoric of sexual purity.

> What is striking therefore is that the white wedding emerged not from any supposed Victorian security over marriage and weddings, but in a period of acute tensions surrounding them. ... The bride and the cake, similarly bedecked, can be seen as a strategy emerging in response to a prevailing situation, marking off the single from the married in typical rite of passage style ... but pushing the sexual implications of the transition well away from the public event itself.
>
> (p. 66)

Charsley considers the situation a hundred years on. By the 1980s everything was different: there was no more secrecy, virginity or indissoluble marriage, and legal reforms in many areas, including benefits and taxation, privileged the individual over the couple or family, in spite of the rhetoric of 'family values'. Marriage had become both of decreasing concern and frequency: 'choice and personal relevance [have] become the new themes'. The arrival of the new technology of sugar paste from Australia allowed for an entirely different style of cake decoration, free of constraints on shape or colour. In this way, Charsley suggests, 'Personalised marriage had finally produced its symbolic counterpart.'

What all the foregoing emphasises, then, is that foods have histories and that practices can only be understood in their historical context. Changes in the wider society – such as new ideas ranging from the relationship between humans and nature, to that between husbands and wives – may be powerfully symbolised by changes in food and eating. Yet continuities may also be discerned – new meanings may be attributed to old practices, or new practices, such as eating out, may incorporate old meanings, such as sociality.

FOOD, DIFFERENCE AND IDENTITY

In his famous gastronomic essay *La Physiologie du gout*, published in 1826, Brillat-Savarin includes the following, oft-quoted aphorism: 'Tell me what you eat and I will tell you who you are.' Somewhat more recently, Fischler, among others, has also argued that food is central to our sense of identity: 'Because we are omnivores, incorporation is an act laden with meaning' (1988: 277). He notes that through the principle of incorporation – 'the action in which we send a food across the frontier between the world and the self, between "outside" and "inside" our body' – we become what we eat (1988: 279). In recent anthropological and sociological work on food and feeding in western societies, there is a preoccupation with food as a marker of difference, including such classic sociological variables as gender, age, class and ethnicity which frequently 'make a difference' to eating patterns, and to which I now turn.

Gender

The question of gender and food is a complex one. In the West, gender is in part a status ascribed by biology, but it is also achieved through 'performance' (Butler 1990, 1994, Moore 1994); this would include not only practices of food and eating, but also the preparation of meals (and the clearing up afterwards).

Thanks to the influence of the feminist movement, there is now a fair amount of information available on food and gender in the West, with several excellent studies: for Britain we have the work of Murcott (1982, 1983, 1995) and Charles and Kerr (1988), for the USA that of DeVault (1991) and for Australia that of Lupton (1996). Strikingly common patterns emerge from these studies. One such is that provisioning and food preparation remain largely the work of women, who are responsible not only for 'feeding the family' but also doing so in a manner which accords with the preferences of its members (especially husbands/male partners), remains within budgetary constraints and is as healthy as possible. DeVault examines the 'language of choice' which masks the frequent deference shown by women to male preferences, or, as Murcott's informants express it: 'It's a pleasure to cook for him' (1983). Men who cook do so less frequently, are more likely to prepare snacks rather than meals, or to cook meals considered particularly appropriate for men: barbecues, Sunday breakfasts or exotic specialities, a point which is also made by Williams in her chapter in this volume.

Second, studies of gender and food often reveal that there are different 'entitlements' to food as between women and men, both in terms of kinds of food and quantity. 'Entitlements' is a term brought into common currency by the economist Amartya Sen in his classic analysis of famines (1981), and later employed both by himself and others as a concept applicable in other contexts too, such as the household (Sen 1990). There may be gender-based differences in entitlements because particular foods are associated with one sex rather than the other. This is particularly notable in the case of meat, which in the West is widely linked to masculinity. 'Real men' are thought to need meat, particularly red meat, as most of the above-cited studies show, and as Bourdieu (1986), Chapman (1990) and Delphy (1979) have demonstrated for France, and Fiddes (1991) and Ellis (1983) for Britain. Conversely vegetarians are much more likely to be female than male (Fiddes 1991, Willetts this volume). Men may also have much greater entitlement than women to alcohol as has been shown by Chapman for France (1990) and Gofton for Britain (1983). A number of studies (Brannen and Wilson 1987, DeVault 1991, Charles and Kerr 1988, Lupton 1996) also suggest that men in the West are entitled to greater quantities of food than women, a pattern with long-established historical precedents in Britain (Pember Reeves 1979, Ross 1994) as in other areas of the world. Furthermore, women as mothers are the ones expected to practise 'maternal altruism' (Whitehead 1981) towards both their children and their male partners, and deny themselves food if there is not enough to go round, again a finding reported in the studies cited above by Charles and Kerr, Murcott, DeVault and Lupton, as well as in a recent study of British women on low incomes by Lobstein (1991).

A third area in which gender is particularly significant in western society is that of dieting and eating disorders, on which there is now an enormous literature, mainly medical and psychological. Women are much more likely to be on weight-reducing diets than men, and are also much more likely to develop eating disorders such as anorexia nervosa or bulimia nervosa. This is a complex and fascinating area with which I do not have space to deal in this introduction, except to note that here we see the ambiguity of powerlessness, on the one hand, in terms of the over-determination of women's body shapes by outside forces, and on the other, power through control not only over appetite but also over social relationships, particularly those of the family (see for example Chernin 1986, Welbourne and Purgold 1984, Lawrence 1984, 1987, Orbach 1986, Hesse-Biber 1991, Bordo 1993, MacSween 1995). Questions of eating disorders are intimately linked to gendered notions of identity and subjectivity, and to conceptions of the body and health.

Class and status

The second area of difference with which I am concerned and which is marked by food is that of class and status, and I make the assumption that in this respect both class-specific subcultures as well as levels of income are significant. There is a long tradition of concern with food in studies of both affluence and poverty in the West.[3] Thorstein Veblen's *Theory of the Leisure Class* (1953), originally published in 1899, and Norbert Elias's *The Civilising Process* (1978 [1939]) both pertain to the former topic, while Seebohm Rowntree's various studies of poverty in Britain, with the first appearing in 1901, and Maud Pember Reeves's *Round About a Pound a Week* (1979 [1913]) are examples of the latter. As we shall see, these traditions have recently been revived by modern researchers building on some of this earlier work. Mennell (1987) and Finkelstein (1985, 1989) both discuss Elias's notion of the 'civilising of appetite', while Stitt and colleagues have utilised Rowntree's dietary in their work on the increasing extent of primary food poverty in Britain (Stitt and Grant 1995, Stitt 1996).

In his book *Distinction* (1986 [1979]) Bourdieu, building upon the ideas of Veblen and Elias, suggests that the upper classes use food, just as they use taste in music, art or clothes, to differentiate themselves from the lower ones. The latter, however, seek to emulate the former, and thus in order to preserve status differences, the upper classes change their tastes again and again. Mintz's (1985) description of the history of sugar in relation to class in Britain illustrates this point very well. So too does Fitchen's (1988) work in the USA on the poor and their desire to be 'Americans first' in terms of their eating habits, even as the wealthier members of society maintain that they should have 'cheese not steak':

Steak for the poor is a notable transgression because it violates the idea that the poor are different from the rest of us; it mocks our sense of societal order that demands separation of rich and poor.

(Fitchen 1988: 330–1)

Aronson's (1982) study of social definitions of entitlement in Britain and the USA between 1885 and 1920 shows how changing power relations between conflicting social groups were reflected in changing definitions of food needs, as science, in the form of nutrition, was used as a rhetorical arena. The recent work of Stitt and colleagues has also considered various dietaries drawn up by a number of bodies for the poor and the very poor in terms of differential entitlements to food; here it is plain that differences are not only about quantity and nutritional quality, but also about palatability and variety (Stitt 1996).

In this volume, James considers the issue of class and status in Britain as a form of difference symbolised by food. She examines representations of British and foreign food, noting that although there has been a rapid process of 'creolisation' in recent years, particularly with the rise of pizza and kebab houses, Chinese and Indian take-aways, and the increase in convenience foods available in supermarkets which draw upon other culinary traditions, there has also been a revival of local and regional gastronomies. She suggests that the latter trend marks the resurrection or revival of food abandoned by the gentry in the eighteenth and nineteenth centuries when they turned to French cuisine, but notes that it remains primarily a high-status, high-priced food:

> Such foods were only to be enjoyed by the few rather than the many, which means that the twin embrace of foreign food and traditional foods were simply recreating, reordering or sustaining old social divisions along class and educational lines.
>
> (p. 81)

Thus, class and status differences may continue to be expressed, although perhaps in a rather more subtle way. James even suggests that eating foreign food may thus now have become a lower-class marker and eating British food a higher one: 'It is, after all, the fact of difference which really makes a difference' (p. 81).

Ethnicity

A third area of difference symbolised by food is ethnicity. Here, although it would appear axiomatic from the literature that national, regional, linguistic and religious distinctions are often marked in culinary fashion, the amount of empirical information on the extent to which ethnicity is relevant in food choice is relatively small and, for Britain, almost non-existent (although Williams's recent work on Welsh foods is significant here (1996)). Rather more research has been carried out in the United States, such as a project on food in three American communities – Italian Americans, black Americans and Native Americans – directed by Mary Douglas (1984). Goode *et al.* show how meal formats and meal cycles among Italian Americans reflect both change and continuity (1984). Theophano and Curtis (1991), utilising the same research, discuss relations between sisters, mothers and daughters in terms of food exchange and reciprocity, showing how the Italian-American community distinguishes and utilises two kinds of meals: those based on traditional Italian cooking (termed 'gravy and one-pot') and American 'platter' meals (similar to the 'meat, potatoes and two vegetables' of British food) which contrast with this.

Similarly, in this volume, Bradby notes that young women of Punjabi origin in Glasgow categorise foods into 'your foods' and 'our foods', and that they eat both, although the evening meal is more likely to consist of foods of the latter category. This finding supports Koctürk-Runefors's (1991) contention that it is in food events which are least symbolically significant that change is likely to take place first. Her suggestion that breakfast will be the first meal to change follows Douglas's contention that it is the least important meal of the daily cycle (1975), and is borne out by the fact that both Italians in North America (Goode *et al.* 1984) and Punjabis in Glasgow (Bradby, this volume) have adopted cereals for breakfast, which represents a considerable shift from previous patterns.

In this volume, Harbottle considers the issue of ethnic identity and food among Iranians in Britain, many of whom have entered the fast food business, in part at least because of the difficulties they have experienced, in spite of their high levels of education, in obtaining jobs in the formal sector. She notes that other immigrants, such as Italians, South Asians and Chinese, have also entered the catering trade, and they have changed British tastes in so doing. There is, however, no such impact with Iranian food since mostly the Iranian outlets sell kebabs, pizzas and burgers, and even the first of these, which the Iranians feel are 'Iranian food', are marketed in the knowledge that British consumers think they are Turkish. Iranians usually do not reveal their national identity at work, since they are well aware that for most British, the resonances of everything Iranian are stigmatising; they prefer to be categorised as southern Europeans. In this way, Iranians feel that they can protect and disguise their identity, not allowing 'their food' to be treated with contempt.

An examination of food and ethnicity must not, of course, content itself with 'ethnic minorities'; it must also interrogate the categories of the dominant majority. In a recent article, Keane and Willetts (1995) note that most of their London informants thought that there was no longer any such thing as British food, and many pointed to the adoption of foreign food items. In her article here, James notes that, paradoxically, Britishness may continue to be marked out in the appearance and ready acceptance of creolised food, provided that it is amenable to the traditional British concerns with saving time and money, and caters to the national sweet tooth; both of these concerns are also reflected in much of the food eaten by tourists in Wales, as discussed in Williams's paper in this volume. In other words, here we have examples of trends unnoticed by most of those who participate in them, scarcely surprising when it is appreciated that the ethnic majority is the *unmarked* category, the Self, rather than the Other, and thus their food is itself deemed to be unremarkable.

FRAGMENTED IDENTITY: THE SUBJECT, THE BODY AND AGENCY

The concept of identity has been questioned on several grounds. One is that it risks essentialising notions such as gender, race, ethnicity and nationality. The counter-argument here is one concerning the 'politics of location' which avers that such concepts do 'make a difference' and that this has important political implications. Furthermore, as Hall points out, such concepts may have been deconstructed, but they have not been replaced: 'The line which cancels them paradoxically permits them to go on being read' since while they may be ideas which cannot be thought in the old way, without them certain questions cannot be thought at all (1995: 1–2).

In his now celebrated book on the risk society (1992 [1986]), Beck argues that the relevance and meaning of such constructs as class, gender and ethnicity have shifted in recent years as we move towards the 'risk society'. He notes the growth in individualism, the reflexive creation of the individual biography made necessary by the forms of today's labour markets with their 'flexible' workforce. Identity now comes as much from 'lifestyle' as it does from the classic sociological concepts of gender, class and race/ethnicity discussed above. This may help to explain Willetts's somewhat puzzling finding, reported in her chapter in this volume, that the majority of her self-defined vegetarian interviewees actually eat meat sometimes. At the BAAS conference at which she delivered her original paper, this aroused enormous media interest. Newspaper reports subsequently appeared under such headlines as 'Bacon tempts most veggies' (*Daily Telegraph* 13.9.95: 4) and 'Vegetarians succumb to a bacon sandwich' (*The Times* 13.9.95: 6). In actuality, it appears to matter less whether or not vegetarians sometimes eat meat, than that people define themselves as vegetarians in the first place as part of their individual identity.[4]

The concept of identity is closely related to others which have been around for longer in anthropology – the person and the self. As Brian Morris notes, cross-cultural understandings of the person have a long history going back to Mauss, Hallowell and Fortes, while more recently, 'self' and 'subjectivity' have also become key concepts in social theory (1994: 1). Yet in adopting such a view, we must not lose sight of the *socially* constructed nature of identity, which is symbolised so clearly by food and commensality: identity cannot be reduced simply to 'lifestyle', or thought of in purely individual terms.

In her recent book on food and the body, Lupton (1996) suggests that post-structuralist approaches generally privilege the notion of the fragmented and contingent rather than the unified self. They have tended to adopt the term 'subjectivity' which is a less rigid one than identity as it incorporates the notion that the self/selves are highly changeable and contextual, albeit within certain limits imposed by culture, including power relations, social institutions and hegemonic discourses. Subjectivity includes an interest in conscious and unconscious thoughts and emotions and the interaction of these with the constitution of the subject through language and discourse.

In this volume, Cohn's work speaks to this approach. He notes that until recently much anthropology has been dominated by symbolic approaches which have removed the individual actor from view. But more recently, there has been increasing concern with the individual in the real world and a rejection of the western notion of a rational, a priori self divorced from lived experience. As Csordas has suggested in his book on the body (1994), the stress on existence as experience places the self as part of the world and the challenge is to recognise that humans are reflexive. Cohn argues that such an approach owes much both to the influence of Heidegger, whose hermeneutics recognised the importance of social influence, as well as to psychoanalytic theory. His paper shows how a diabetic patient talks to a medical professional and to the ethnographer about her illness, suggesting ways in which meanings are interpreted and lived out, rather than passively accepted, in spite of the dominance of the medical script. Her conversation with the ethnographer demonstrates how the idea of the illness is related to a concept of the self as experienced in her life activity beyond the Diabetes Day Centre.

At the same time, as Lupton and others have pointed out, a post-structuralist, indeed, postmodern approach has increasingly incorporated the body into its focus. The human body is seen as a project, an entity in the process of becoming, dynamic not static, and subject to conscious moulding. Utilising Foucault's ideas on the 'practices' or 'technologies' of the self, Lupton notes that they 'represent the site at which discourses and physical phenomena may be adopted as part of the individual's project to construct and express subjectivity' (1996: 15). Such practices 'inscribe' or 'write' on the body which is then 'read' or interpreted by others.

The modern 'retreat into the body' means that it has become highly constitutive of the self; as a result, negative events which befall it constitute a frightening challenge to subjectivity (Shilling 1993). For this reason, illness and even death are now viewed as failures of the self, and indications of a lack of rational behaviour and self-control, especially around issues of food and eating which are central practices of the self. Thus, in an age of uncertainty and heightened self-reflexivity, one way of taking control over the body is to exert discipline over eating habits. Given the current value of 'self-control', bodies become potent physical symbols of the extent to which their 'owners' possess self-control.

However, such generalising theories are insufficient to explain the complexity of concepts around food and the body, and need to be accompanied by empirical qualitative research. Keane and Willetts's work in South-East London suggests that interviewees stress their embodied individuality (Keane and Willetts 1995, Keane, forthcoming). Informants there spoke continuously of 'my body and what's good for me', and many also mentioned 'listening to their bodies', or, as Cohn puts it in his chapter, 'the body talks'. In her chapter in this book, Keane makes use of the concept of 'embodied knowledge' as a way of discussing how participants in her study privilege their own experience concerning food and health above other sources of information.

Some postmodern approaches are insufficient to explain the complexity of concepts regarding food and the body, and can, as Hall points out in his recent volume on identity (1995), be in danger of leaving out vital questions of agency and power. Hall argues that we do not need an abandonment or abolition of 'the subject' but a reconceptualisation which incorporates agency, intention and volition. This may be a useful way of reading Finkelstein's work on dining, in which she suggests that what is eaten and where makes dining out an eloquent index of social value, a symbol of civility (1985, 1989). She takes her notion of civility from Elias and defines it as 'a social relation in which the individual does not act ego-centrically or absent-mindedly, but rather is aware of a surrounding culture and a predisposing history' (1985: 184). Her argument is that dining out has become, in the late twentieth century, an act of failed civility because of what she terms 'high consumerism' and the modernist fragmentation of the self: 'the rampant consumerism of individuals in the industrialized nations . . . demonstrates . . . the transformation of all that is held valuable into material objects' (1985: 205). Yet to some extent, her arguments had already been anticipated and rebutted by Douglas:

The ordinary consuming public in modern industrial society works hard to invest its food with moral, social and aesthetic meanings. The actual current meaningfulness of food is being overlooked by professional food theorists because their thought is doubly restricted, partly by antique metaphysical assumptions about the separation of spirit and flesh and partly by an intellectual tradition which has desocialized the individual.

(1984: 5)

In this volume, Martens and Warde likewise take issue with Finkelstein's portrayal of the hedonistic, unthinking and uncaring diner-out. In their study of eating out in a northern city in Britain, they found that people can be perfectly articulate about their likes and dislikes: they enjoy the pleasure of anticipation, trying new foods, escaping from domestic labour. They see eating out as 'special', and this is dependent upon it being an occasional activity. Even in situations where the quality or ambience is poor, they are willing to balance this against the positive factors of sociability and having a night out with friends. Diners are seen as actively participating in and shaping the event: 'In general, people are discerning, self-conscious and aware of the various elements of the experience of eating out and can thus talk about them in discriminating fashion' (pp. 148–9). In short, they perceive their informants as agents.

A similar set of arguments applies to the way in which people understand the relationship between food and health.

FOOD AND HEALTH

Flowing on from recent changes in western eating habits is an increasing preoccupation with the health effects of the modern high-fat and high-sugar diet, lamented by numerous nutritional and official reports (e.g. HEC 1983, DHSS 1984, Secretary of State for Health 1992). The government response for the last couple of decades has been to encourage 'healthy eating' as part of 'consumer choice' (Secretary of State for Health 1992, Nutrition Task Force 1994).[5] Nonetheless, as Keane points out in this volume, the evidence suggests that this campaign has not had much effect on actual decisions made about what people buy and eat, in spite of the fact that most studies indicate that people are well aware of what constitutes 'healthy food' according to current nutritional wisdom. Keane's review of healthy eating policies argues that the official perception of such information as straightforward 'facts' which the public can choose to accept or ignore has to be questioned, since the government exhorts consumers to choose healthy food, while leaving industry to regulate itself. She states that 'healthy eating is clearly a political issue' and that most information about food and health is driven, whether implicitly or explicitly, by commercial considerations.

Much research has noted that people are sceptical of current health education messages because they do not seem to correspond with their own experience. A good example is a study by Davison and colleagues of official attempts to prevent chronic disease through encouraging behavioural change, especially in diet. Davison's research was based in South Wales, an area of Britain which has one of the highest rates of heart disease in the United Kingdom and where 'Heartbeat Wales', a division of the Welsh Health Promotion Authority, has carried out an extensive and high-profile campaign.[6] A large part of its work is built on the slogan of 'choosing health', with the implication that 'much heart disease is attributable either to ignorance, or to a lack of self-discipline' (Davison *et al.* 1991: 3). Davison and his colleagues discuss a well-developed lay epidemiology which enables people to assess the risks of their eating behaviour. A prime concern is that of candidacy:

A mechanism that helps individuals to assess personal risks, obtain reassuring affirmation of predictability, identify the limits of that predictability . . . devise appropriate strategies of personal behaviour and to go some way towards explaining events which, by their very nature, are deeply distressing.

(1991: 6)

Many of the behaviours which are incorporated into the candidacy system are aspects of life which are seen as open to *choice*, yet at the same time, there is a risk of 'blaming the victim'. On the other hand, as with all such explanations, there is a built-in failure mechanism – the system is recognised to be fallible through the element of *chance*, with heart disease also being seen as a random killer. Elsewhere, Davison explains this in terms of two important figures. On the one hand, there are the 'Uncle Normans', as in 'my uncle Norman ate bacon and eggs every day and lived till 93'. On the other, there are those who are seen as 'the last person you'd expect', for example, to have a coronary. So while people know that fatty food is bad for you, they also know that this is not always the case. They live, after all, in a complex landscape of relative risk and are thus led both to believe and disbelieve the health food messages. Scarcely surprising, then, that so many people in Britain today are 'sceptical eaters' and see little point in changing their diets (Davison 1989).

In a subsequent article (Davison *et al.* 1992), the same authors consider the issue of risk, which has become a central concept in both lay and professional discourse in the late twentieth century, partly, they suggest, because of the change from acute to chronic diseases. They develop further their notion of a lay epidemiology, which, while acknowledging the importance of lifestyle, utilises in addition a recognition of such collective and environmental forces as heredity, wealth and occupation which are outside of individual control.

Davison *et al.* suggest that people deal with such factors through a concept of fatalism which incorporates a number of lay notions, including, *inter alia*, religion ('the will of the Almighty'), and the 'allotted lifespan'. Such ideas attempt to explain not only the how and why of illness and death, but also why this particular person is afflicted at this point in time, a perhaps more important question to which Evans-Pritchard drew attention in his classic anthropological study of African witchcraft (1937). Davison *et al.* maintain that one of the reasons why people find the official discourse on health so unsatisfying is that it attempts to reduce the second kind of question (why me? why now?) to a sub-set of the first (how and why). Indeed, the official discourse on healthy eating actually utilises epidemiological findings ('risk', probability) as if they were causal explanations. Lay epidemiology, on the other hand, is much more critical.

Further articles by Backett and Davison (1992), and Backett *et al.* (1994) compare the South Wales data with studies carried out in Scotland, revealing several important commonalities in their findings. The first is that the respondents perceived a very wide variety of influences on health and illness, not just that of lifestyle. Second, respondents in all areas were sceptical about scientific information because they saw it as changing from time to time. Third, people utilised an active health management strategy by adopting what they saw as 'reasonable' courses of action in terms of costs and benefits. They practised 'trade-offs' in terms of eating healthily versus unhealthily, well aware that risky behaviour can be life-enhancing even while it is not health-enhancing, but justifying their actions through the useful concepts of 'moderation' and 'balance'. Elsewhere, Backett and Davison (1992) note that what is considered to be reasonable behaviour is itself context-dependent, focusing particularly upon stages of the life-cycle which 'implies having different priorities about behaviour relevant to health', including eating (1992).

The findings in Keane's chapter in this book have much in

common with those of Davison and colleagues. For her South-East London interviewees, information was viewed as coming from a generalised 'they' which included scientists, the medical profession, journalists and promoters of new diets. The media were seen as sensationalist and alarmist in their coverage of food issues. Informants maintained a stance of scepticism to healthy-eating advice, castigating it as biased to commercial interests, and complaining that they were not given enough information about issues such as additives or genetic and environmental processes which concerned them more and were often seen as more important than healthy eating. In any case, general information was often not thought to be relevant to specific situations since all informants considered individual variability of crucial importance.

Keane identified age and gender differences in relation to adherence to healthy-eating advice from different sources. While older people were likely to view their GPs as authoritative sources of advice, younger interviewees tended to shop around for information. They consulted health professionals for nutritional advice only under specific circumstances – women when pregnant, parents about their young children, males when middle-aged – and otherwise said they mistrusted professional advice. They did, however, take notice of what friends and relatives said, particularly because such information came in the form of a dialogue, and was also seen as more relevant to other aspects of daily life.

A similar scepticism towards medical advice on nutrition was evinced by the patients in a diabetic clinic studied by Cohn (Chapter 10 this volume). The treatment offered here usually fails: patients expect medication from doctors, not dietary advice, and they accord it less significance than tablets or insulin. For patients, lifestyle advice is seen as more open to review, and food to be within the personal and social, not medical domain. In any case, keeping to the lifestyle advice in a way which would satisfy the medical profession means at the same time acknowledging an enduring sick identity, a stance which patients are highly reluctant to adopt.

It is thus scarcely surprising that in spite of medical advice, many patients continue, for example, to perceive sugar as central to their diet, symbolising as it does both pleasure and necessity, and playing an important role in maintaining balance within a model based on an underlying theme of labour and consumption. Thus, as Cohn notes, having a treat 'is a recognition and an affirmation of the self as it always has been, a self not betrayed by others, with the usual routines, usual requirements and usual balance' (p. 209).

Williams's paper on food on holiday, with data gathered from tourists in South-West Wales, also examines the notion of the 'treat'. Her interviewees made frequent contrasts between the way they eat at home and on holiday. Being away from home meant that the usual boundaries between normal and abnormal food are weaker than usual, and people 'confessed' to succumbing to 'horrendous hamburgers', chips or 'cream teas'. However, it may be mistaken to view such eating as a lapse or transgression, even though the discourses are frequently redolent with moral judgements, because most people recognise that being on holiday is different: their labour for the rest of the year entitles them to change the (usually healthy) eating rules, and eat primarily for pleasure. In this way, cycles of 'control' (home) versus 'release' (holiday) not only make the former more acceptable, but the latter, by their relative infrequency, more enjoyable. Because the latter cycle takes place in a defined space and time, it does not threaten the rules of the former.

Williams notes that in talking about food on holiday, interviewees were often, either implicitly or explicitly, also talking about food at home, drawing contrasts not only in terms of items consumed, but also in terms of moral rules, often predicated upon a distinction between 'good (enjoyable) food' and '(healthy) food which is good for you', a distinction which has been noted in a number of studies (e.g. Murcott 1995).

RISK AND REFLEXIVITY

A number of recent studies of food in the West draw upon wider studies of risk perception, particularly the work of Douglas (Douglas and Wildavsky 1982, Douglas 1992) and Beck (1992, originally published in German in 1986). Douglas and Wildavsky note that in recent years, confidence in the physical world has increasingly turned into doubt. While much of the research on risk perception has been done by psychologists, it is their argument that the choice of risks with which people are concerned is first and foremost socially determined. Beck maintains that discourses about risk and distribution of risks are becoming central themes of society and argues that risk consciousness is more likely to develop when direct pressures to make a living, to achieve the basic necessities of food and shelter, are no longer present to the same degree as formerly. Further, it is Beck's contention that our situation when confronted by hazards is essentially the same regardless of background variables; risks today concern everyone. Beck develops the notion of what he terms 'reflexive modernity', a situation in which people attempt to reconcile different priorities with regard to risk issues and are highly sceptical of the progressive claims of modernity and science.

Work on risk has been influential in material on food published in the 1990s (e.g. Fürst *et al.* 1991). A study by Lupton and Chapman (1995) of discourses on diet, cholesterol control and heart disease in the press and among the lay public in Australia suggests that here, too, late modernity is characterised by increasing focus on anxiety about risk, including that to health. Assessment of risk may require medical advice, but individuals also weigh up risks using personal experience and lay knowledge. In this way health promotional orthodoxies are subject to continued negotiation and challenge on the part of members of the public.

There is some evidence that a significant number of people do seek to bring some control into their lives by adopting a particular dietary and exercise regime. But none of the advice on, for example, cutting down on fats on the grounds that over-consumption increases the risk of coronary heart disease, has had anything like the effect on consumer choice as has been occasioned by such food 'scares' as salmonella in eggs or bovine spongiform encephalopathy in cattle. Frankel *et al.* (1991) compare the worries about eggs in terms of both cholesterol and salmonella, suggesting that these represent two different kinds of risk. In the first, which they label 'bad but desirable', the risks are not immediate, and are often counter-balanced by explicit benefits, such as enjoyment. The second kind of risk is the 'bad/poisonous' category. Here, for example, the eggs are seen to be contaminated by a pathogen which speedily produces very unpleasant effects. The 'poison' can, however, be conceptually separated from the food itself, thus restoring the food to a benign state. This is an oversimplified taxonomy since the categories are constantly shifting, often by design: advertisers seek to move food which is bad/dangerous into the category of bad/desirable (naughty but nice), while popular jokes seek to ensure that desirable foods and drinks remain in the latter, not the former category ('What's your poison?').

There is no doubt that the issue of risk and risk perception is a highly political one, as Reilly and Miller's chapter in this volume on the media and the BSE crisis makes clear. They show how the way in which a crisis such as BSE is presented in the media is a complex and far from homogeneous or predictable process. The media themselves are differentiated and are dependent upon their information sources. In effect, the media provide an arena of contestation. Furthermore, their impact upon the public depends upon a number of factors external to the media themselves.

The British government, particularly MAFF (Ministry of Agriculture, Fisheries and Food) has been concerned to lay issues of food risk at the door of the individual consumer, hence the plethora of 'healthy eating' advice. For example, the salmonella scare in 1988–9 was precipitated by the public admission of the then Junior Health Minister Edwina Currie that 'most of the egg production of this country, sadly, is now infected with salmonella'. There is evidence that the salmonella concerned (Entiritidis Phage type 4), unlike other salmonellas, is linked less to poor kitchen hygiene than to intensive poultry-rearing systems. Nonetheless, the government response to the crisis brought about by an overnight drop of 50 per cent in egg sales was, Reilly and Miller note, a 'shift of perceptions from egg production to kitchen hygiene' (p. 237, see also Macdonald and Silverstone 1992).

Reilly and Miller then go on to discuss the BSE food panic, noting that until March 1996 official statements insisted that it posed no risk to humans. They show how MAFF had earlier managed to keep public health interests out of the decision-making process in a number of ways: by stressing that BSE was a veterinary problem, by attempting to control which experts were deemed to be such, and by influencing what people were allowed to say in public. At that point however, the Minister of Health announced the existence of a new strain of CJD (Creutzfeld-Jakob disease to which humans are subject) which was probably linked to BSE; this statement changed the nature of the BSE debate, and also resulted in the European ban on British beef.

In an earlier publication (1991) Fiddes has argued that what a whole range of food scares have in common is that they are perceived as 'unnatural': feeding the carcasses of dead chickens to others, or the remains of sheep to cattle as part of commercial cattle feed is seen as tampering with nature in an unacceptable way. Chickens are not supposed to be cannibalistic, nor are cattle carnivores. Furthermore, British people do not eat carnivores. Thus modern feeding and production methods are seen to be particularly unacceptable when they cause animals used for food to move out of their normal categories, an argument which harks back to the already-cited early work of Mary Douglas (1966).

CONCLUSION: AGENCY, VOLITION AND INTENTIONALITY

This chapter has shown that recent changes in food and eating cannot be summarily dismissed as symptomatic only of alienation and anomie. Rather, as the articles in this book suggest, people continue actively to construct meanings around the food they consume: they develop taxonomies, articulate satisfaction or dissatisfaction with food, resist advertising or medical messages, and in this respect they are agents. This does not mean, of course, that issues of power can be ignored but it can be resisted as well as accepted, and this is seen in a variety of ways in relation to food. 'Healthy-eating' advice may be rejected because of a lay epidemiology which deems it inappropriate or unreasonable. People may attempt to control the process of incorporation of risky food through adopting particular diets, demanding more information, joining pressure groups or simply refusing to purchase items which they deem unsafe.

If, then, we are to make sense of food and eating in the West today, particularly in Britain, we need to understand not only a variety of social, cultural and historical contexts, but also the many layers of knowledge and meaning held by different subjects, and even by a single subject, in relation to food and eating. Such knowledge is both socially and culturally constructed, as well as being developed by particular subjects in terms of their own identities, their life histories and their views of themselves and their bodies. We need, then, to see food consumers both as agents, imbued with volition and intentionality, and as social beings, continuing to use food to express significant relationships. It is our hope that this collection goes some way towards meeting these needs.

NOTES

1 Apart from the publication of Richards's much praised but little emulated 1939 study of food among the Bemba, a people of central

Africa, food did not really become a fashionable topic in British anthropology until the 1960s.
2 Considerable amounts of work on food and historical change have been carried out by historians, notably Camporesi for Italy (1989 and 1993), Braudel and the *Annales* school for France and other parts of Europe (Braudel 1985, Forster and Ranum 1979), Drummond and Wilbraham (1991 [1939]) and Burnett (1983 [1966]) for Britain, and Mennell (1985) for England and France, to mention only some of the more notable examples.
3 It is a curious paradox that even as social inequalities in western societies, especially Britain, increase, most people lack a vocabulary with which to discuss this phenomenon. Many social scientists, having jettisoned the notion of class, find themselves in a similar position to the lay public, and in this respect, have perhaps colluded with the makers of policies which have increased the divide.
4 In a personal communication, Hannah Bradby suggests that it is only when bodies are liberated from the daily grind of poverty, and in cultures where there is not a strong system of religion or honour, that 'lifestyle' begins to play a role in food choice. A lifestyle in which one chooses to become a vegetarian suggests a great fluidity and manipulability of the symbolism of food. This fluidity may not exist for marginalised groups.
5 There is a plethora of 'healthy-eating' pamphlets, leaflets and posters put out by the Health Education Authority, the Ministry of Agriculture Fisheries and Food, the Department of Health, and local Health Authorities, as well as specific campaigns such as: 'Look after your heart'. In addition, many food retailers produce 'healthy-eating' leaflets, and in recent years, government bodies have often combined with food retailers to produce material jointly.
6 Hybu Lechyd Cymru/Health Promotion Wales has run numerous campaigns, and produced many reports which are listed in their 1996 catalogue.

REFERENCES

Aronson, N. (1982) 'Social definitions of entitlement; food needs 1885–1920', *Media Culture & Society* 4, 4: 57–61.
Backett, K. and Davison, C. (1992) 'Rational or reasonable? Perceptions of health at different stages of life', *Health Education Journal* 51: 55–9.
Backett, K., Davison, C. and Mullen, K. (1994) 'Lay evaluation of health and healthy lifestyles: evidence from three studies', *British Journal of General Practice* 44: 277–80.
Barthes, R. (1975) 'Towards a psychosociology of contemporary food consumption', in E. Forster and R. Forster (eds) *European Diet from Pre-industrial to Modern Times*, New York: Harper Row.
Beck, U. (1992) [1986] *Risk Society: Towards a New Modernity*, London: Sage Publications.

Bordo, S. (1993) *Unbearable Weight: Feminism, Western Culture and the Body*, Berkeley: University of California Press.

Bourdieu, P. (1986) [1979] *Distinction: A Social Critique of the Judgement of Taste*, London: Routledge and Kegan Paul.

Brannen, J. and Wilson, G. (eds) (1987) *Give and Take in Families: Studies in Resource Distribution*, London: Allen and Unwin.

Braudel, F. (1985) [1979] *Civilization and Capitalism, 15th–18th Centuries*, London: Fontana.

Burnett, John (1983) [1966] *Plenty and Want: A Social History of Diet in England from 1815 to the Present Day*, London: Methuen.

Butler, J. (1990) *Gender Trouble: Feminism and the Subversion of Identity*, New York, London: Routledge.

—— (1994) *Bodies that Matter*, New York and London: Routledge.

Camporesi, P. (1989) [1980] *Bread of Dreams: Food and Fantasy in Early Modern Europe*, Cambridge: Polity Press.

—— (1993) *The Magic Harvest: Food, Folklore and Society*, Cambridge: Polity Press.

Chapman, G. and Maclean, H. (1993) '"Junk food" and "healthy food": meanings of food in adolescent women's culture', *Journal of Nutrition Education* 25, 3: 108–13.

Chapman, M. (1990) 'The social definition of want', in M. Chapman and H. Macbeth (eds) *Food for Humanity: Cross-disciplinary Readings*, Oxford: Oxford Polytechnic.

Charles, N. and Kerr, M. (1988) *Women, Food and Families*, Manchester: Manchester University Press.

Charsley, S. (1992) *Wedding Cakes and Cultural History*, London: Routledge.

Chernin, K. (1986) *The Hungry Self: Women, Eating and Identity*, London: Virago Press.

Csordas, T. (ed.) (1994) *Embodiment and Experience: The Existential Ground of Culture and Self*, Cambridge: Cambridge University Press.

Davison, C. (1989) 'Eggs and the sceptical eater', *New Scientist* 11 March: 45–9.

Davison, C., Frankel, S. and Smith, G.D. (1992) 'The limits of life-style: reassessing "fatalism" in the popular culture of illness prevention', *Social Science & Medicine* 34: 675–85.

Davison, C., Smith, G.D. and Frankel, S. (1991) 'Lay epidemiology and the prevention paradox: the implications of coronary candidacy for health education', *Social Health & Illness* 13, 1: 1–19.

Delphy, C. (1979) 'Sharing the same table: consumption and the family', in C. Harris (ed.) *The Sociology of the Family: New Directions for Britain*, Sociological Review Monograph no. 28, Keele: Keele University Press.

DeVault, M. (1991) *Feeding the Family: The Social Organisation of Caring as Gendered Work*, Chicago: Chicago University Press.

DHSS (Department of Health and Social Security) (1984) *Diet and Cardiovascular Disease: Report of the Committee on the Medical Aspects of Food Policy*, London: COMA/HMSO.

Douglas, M. (1966) 'The abominations of Leviticus', in M. Douglas, *Purity and Danger*, London: Routledge and Kegan Paul.

—— (1975) 'Deciphering a meal', in M. Douglas, *Implicit Meanings*, London: Routledge and Kegan Paul.

—— (1984) *Food in the Social Order: Studies of Food and Festivities in Three American Communities*, New York: Russell Sage Foundation.

—— (1992) *Risk and Blame: Essays in Cultural Theory*, London: Routledge.

Douglas, M. and Nicod, M. (1974) 'Taking the biscuit: the structure of British meals', *New Society* 33: 744–7.

Douglas, M. and Wildavsky, A. (1982) *Risk and Culture: An Essay on the Selection of Technical and Environmental Dangers*, Berkeley and Los Angeles: University of California Press.

Drummond, J. and Wilbraham, A. (1991) [1939] *The Englishman's Food*, London: Pimlico.

Elias, N. (1978) [1939] *The Civilising Process, vol. I: The History of Manners*, Oxford: Blackwell.

Ellis, R. (1983) 'The way to a man's heart: food in the violent home', in A. Murcott (ed.) *The Sociology of Food and Eating*, Swansea: Gower Press.

Evans-Pritchard, E. (1937) *Witchcraft, Oracles and Magic Among the Azande*, Oxford: Clarendon Press.

Falk, P. (1994) *The Consuming Body*, London: Sage.

Fiddes, N. (1991) *Meat: A Natural Symbol*, London and New York: Routledge.

Finkelstein, J. (1985) 'Dining out: the self in search of civility', *Studies in Symbolic Interaction* 6: 183–212.

—— (1989) *Dining Out: A Sociology of Modern Manners*, Cambridge: Polity Press.

Fischler, C. (1980) 'Food habits, social change and the nature/culture dilemma', *Social Science Information* 19: 937–53.

—— (1988) 'Food, self and identity', *Social Science Information* 27, 2: 275–92.

Fitchen, J.M. (1988) 'Hunger, malnutrition and poverty in the contemporary United States: some observations on their social and cultural context', *Food and Foodways* 2: 309–33.

Forster, R. and Ranum, O. (eds) (1979) *Food and Drink in History: Selections from the Annales E.S.C.*, Baltimore: Johns Hopkins University Press.

Frankel, S., Davison, C. and Smith, G.D. (1991) 'Lay epidemiology and the rationality of responses to health education', *British Journal of General Practice* 41: 428–30.

Fürst, E.L., Prättalä, R., Ekström, M., Holm, L. and Kjaernes, V. (eds) (1991) *Palatable Worlds: Sociocultural Food Studies*, Oslo: Solum Forlag.

Gofton, L. (1983) 'Real ale and real men', *New Society* 17 November: 271–3.

Goode, J., Curtis, K. and Theophano, J. (1984) 'Meal formats, meal cycles and menu negotiation in the maintenance of an Italian-American community', in M. Douglas (ed.) *Food in the Social Order*, New York: Russell Sage Foundation.

Goody, J. (1982) *Cooking, Cuisine and Class*, Cambridge: Cambridge University Press.

Hall, S. (1995) 'Who needs identity?' in S. Hall and P. Du Day (eds) *Questions of Cultural Identity*, London: Sage Publications.

Harris, M. (1985) *Good to Eat: Riddles of Food and Culture*, New York: Simon and Schuster.

Harris, M. and Ross, E.B. (1987) *Food and Evolution: Toward a Theory of Human Food Habits*, Philadelphia: Temple University Press.

HEC (Health Education Council) (1983) *A Discussion Paper on Proposals for National Guidelines for Health Education in Britain*, London: NACNE.

Hesse-Biber, S. (1991) 'Women, weight and eating disorders: a socio-cultural and political-economic analysis', *Women's Studies International Forum* 14, 3: 173–92.

James, A. (1982) 'Confections, concoctions and conceptions', in B. Waites, T. Bennett and G. Martin (eds) *Popular Culture: Past and Present*, London: Croom Helm.

Keane, A. (forthcoming) 'Conceptualising food and the self: normality and the body as potential. An anthropological study in South-East London', PhD thesis: University of London.

Keane, A. and Willetts, A. (1995) 'Concepts of healthy eating: An anthropological investigation in South-East London', Working Paper (mimeo), London: Goldsmiths' College.

Koctürk-Runefors, T. (1991) 'A model for adaptation to a new food pattern', in E.L. Fürst, R. Prättala, M. Ekström, L. Holm and V. Kjaernes (eds) *Palatable Worlds: Sociocultural Food Studies*, Oslo: Solum Forlag.

Lawrence, M. (1984) *The Anorexic Experience*, London: The Women's Press.

—— (ed.) (1987) *Fed Up and Hungry: Women, Oppression and Food*, London: The Women's Press.

Leach, E. (1964) 'Anthropological aspects of language: animal categories and verbal abuse', in E.H. Lennenberg (ed.) *New Directions in the Study of Language*, Cambridge, Mass.: MIT Press.

Lévi-Strauss, C. (1965) 'The culinary triangle', *Partisan Review* 33: 586–95.

—— (1968) *Structural Anthropology*, vol. I, Harmondsworth: Allen Lane, Penguin Press.

—— (1970) *The Raw and the Cooked*, New York: Harper Torchbooks.

Lobstein, T. (1991) 'The nutrition of women on low incomes', mimeo, London: The Food Commission.

Lupton, D. (1996) *Food, the Body and the Self*, London: Sage Publications.

Lupton, D. and Chapman, S. (1995) 'A healthy life-style might be the death of you: discourses on diet, cholesterol control and heart disease in the press and among the lay public', *Sociology of Health and Illness* 17, 4: 477–94.

Macdonald, S. and Silverstone, R. (1992) 'Science on display: the representation of scientific controversy in museum exhibitions', *Public Understanding of Science* 1: 69–87.

MacSween, M. (1995) *Anorexic Bodies: A Feminist and Sociological Perspective on Anorexia Nervosa*, London and New York: Routledge.

Mennell, S. (1985) *All Manners of Food: Eating and Taste in England and France from the Middle Ages to the Present*, Oxford: Blackwell.

—— (1987) 'On the civilizing of appetite', *Theory, Culture & Society* 4, 3–4: 373–403.

Mintz, S. (1984) 'Meals without grace', *Boston Review*, December.

—— (1985) *Sweetness and Power: The Place of Sugar in Modern History*, New York: Viking Press.

—— (1992) 'A taste of history', *The Higher* 8 May: 15, 18.

—— (1994) 'Eating and being: what food means', in B. Harris and R. Hoffenberg (eds) *Food: Multidisciplinary Perspectives*, Oxford: Blackwell.

Moore, H. (1994) *A Passion for Difference*, Cambridge: Polity Press.

Morris, B. (1994) *Anthropology of the Self: The Individual in Cultural Perspective*, London: Pluto Press.

Murcott, A. (1982) 'On the social significance of the "cooked dinner" in South Wales', *Social Science Information* 21, 4/5.

—— (1983) '"It's a pleasure to cook for him": food, mealtimes and gender in some South Wales households', in E. Gamarnikow, D. Morgan, J. Purvis and D. Taylorson (eds) *The Public and the Private*, London: Heinemann.

—— (1995) 'Talking of good food: an empirical study of women's conceptualisations', *Food and Foodways* 40: 305–18.

Nutrition Task Force (1994) *Nutrition and Health: A Management Handbook for the NHS*, London: Department of Health.

Orbach, S. (1986) *Hunger Strike: The Anorectic's Struggle as a Metaphor of our Age*, London: Faber and Faber.

Pember Reeves, M. (1979) [1913] *Round About a Pound a Week*, London: Virago.

Richards, A. (1939) *Land, Labour and Diet in Northern Rhodesia*, London: Routledge and Kegan Paul.

Ross, E. (1994) *Love and Toil: Motherhood in Outcast London, 1870–1918*, Oxford: Oxford University Press.

Rowntree, B.S. (1901) *Poverty: A Study of Town Life*, London: Macmillan.

Sahlins, M. (1976) *Culture and Practical Reason*, Chicago: Chicago University Press.

Secretary of State for Health (1992) *The Health of the Nation*, London: HMSO.

Sen, A. (1981) *Poverty and Famines: An Essay on Entitlement and Deprivation*, Oxford: Oxford University Press.

—— (1990) 'Gender and cooperative conflicts', in I. Tinker (ed.) *Persistent Inequalities: Women and World Development*, Oxford: Oxford University Press.

Shilling, C. (1993) *The Body and Social Theory*, London: Sage Publications.

Stitt, S. (1996) 'When health promotion doesn't work: food poverty in the UK', paper for International Conference on Health Promotion and Nutrition, Wageningen, January.

Stitt, S. and Grant, D. (1995) 'Primary food poverty in Britain', in E. Feichtinger and B.N. Köhler (eds) *Current Research into Eating Practices*, Potsdam: AGEV Publication Series vol. 10.

Theophano, J. and Curtis, K. (1991) 'Sisters, mothers and daughters: food exchange and reciprocity in an Italian-American community', in A. Sharman, J. Theophano and K. Curtis (eds) *Diet and Domestic Life in Society*, Philadelphia: Temple University Press.

Veblen, T. (1953) [1899] *The Theory of the Leisure Class*, New York: Merton.

Welbourne, J. and Purgold, J. (1984) *The Eating Sickness: Anorexia, Bulimia and the Myth of Suicide by Slimming*, Brighton: Harvester Press.

Whitehead, A. (1981) '"I'm hungry, Mum": the politics of domestic budgeting', in Kate Young, C. Walkowitz and R. McCullough (eds) *Of Marriage and the Market*, London: CSE Books.

Williams, J. (1996) 'Globalization in rural Wales: some dietary changes and continuities on Welsh farms', Working Paper (mimeo), London: Goldsmiths' College.

Yudkin, J. and McKenzie, J.C. (1964) *Changing Food Habits*, London: MacGibbon and Kee.

Chapter 2

Family meals – a thing of the past?

Anne Murcott

Meal-time as family reunion time was taken for granted a generation ago . . . there is arising a conscious effort to 'save meal-times, at least, for the family.' As one mother expressed it . . . . 'Even if we have only a little time at home together, we want to make the most of that little. In our family we always try to have Sunday breakfast and dinner together at least.' . . . 'I ate only seven meals at home all last week and three of those were on Sunday' said one father.

Over the past 40 years there has been a food revolution in Britain. New foods and new methods of growing, processing, distributing and cooking food have arrived. Even eating has been transformed. No longer does everyone have so-called family meals all seated round a table. We have snacks between meals, buy low nutrient foods and eat on the hoof – appropriately known by the food marketers as 'grazing'.

[I]t is worrying that . . . breaking bread together is no longer the focal point of family life; a snatched breakfast – if any – being followed by lunch at school or work, with the evening meal a matter of individually finding what is available and gobbling it up in front of the telly . . . or perhaps hunger is assuaged at a fish and chip shop or the ubiquitous McDonalds.

There are probably few surprises in this trio of quotations (their sources are provided later in the chapter). Talk of the changes reputedly under way, the attempts made to resist them, the apprehension at the supposed speed of change and/or its inexorability are, no doubt, quite familiar. Journalists writing on the state of society today, family life or childhood in crisis, use it to signal a disappearing reference point, a shorthand to convey a sense of history, a metaphor for some period or other that has passed.[1] Sociologists and social anthropologists too have assumed the family meal is in decline. For Claude Fischler, it is a case of 'gastro-anomie' (Fischler 1979) – without rules for meal-taking, we are left normless, without guidance. Sidney Mintz, never apparently persuaded that rules were so essential in the first place, nevertheless assumes meal patterns are collapsing (Mintz 1985: 200–4) as does Pasi Falk (1994). Familiar too, is the likelihood that such trends are talked of not as grounds for celebration but reason for alarm and disapproval. Family meals, it is said, are on the wane, rapidly and worryingly becoming a thing of the past.

This chapter revolves around claims such as these. Its main concern, however, is not to assess the rate of the supposed decline, or debate the reasons for it. Instead, a key interest is in reflection on, and speculation about, the very fact that anyone supposes that family meals are on the wane. In part, then, the concern also has to be with evidence – or, more accurately, with discussing types of evidence. On what evidence do commentators declare that the family meal is in decline? Is that evidence strong enough to bear the weight of their conclusions? If not, what kinds of evidence should we be looking for? What phenomena do we need evidence about? These and more are the kind of consideration that this chapter suggests needs to be taken up. In the process, the chapter inevitably has to pay some attention to definitions – so doing is integral to examining evidence. Like it or not, there are times when, however infuriating an academic tic it may seem, the proper first reaction has to be 'it all depends what you mean by . . .' and proceed from there. What kind of family? What kind of worry?[2]

Before outlining what is to come, one or two observations are needed about what this chapter is and is not seeking to accomplish. While it does deal with evidence, the chapter does not represent an exhaustive or comprehensive review of the data even though (assuming the evidence is available) the task of systematically drawing it together, soberly weighing up its dependability and deciding on its interpretation apparently still remains to be done. Indeed, the chapter is not a review at all, but a set of general thoughts that would need to precede the writing of such a review.

What follows is divided into two main sections. The first examines some realities. What data are available about whether people really do or do not have family meals now compared to some earlier period? Is there evidence about whether they subscribe to some idea of family meals, no matter what their actual eating arrangements might be? If so is it an idea to be cherished or disdained? The second main section revisits a little history but shifts the focus to consider the reality of the family meal from different angles. It asks about the kind of family in question, and does so as a way of reflecting on the source of the idea of family meals. And last, it returns to ponder on the very fact that claims are made, and worries expressed, about the waning of the family meal.

IMAGES, REALITIES AND ASPIRATIONS

Amongst the young mothers of pre-school children in Charles and Kerr's (1988) well-known survey, a family meal is readily described and highly valued:

> everybody will sit down together and take time over eating a meal.

> [we all] sit down with a knife and fork and there's potatoes and meat and veg and whatever . . . the main meal of the day that.

> I think they are very, very important because I think it's the time when the family come together, and it's really the only time they come together as a family. Which is why we all sit down and have a chance to talk.

> Very important, it's part of the family existence, it's one of the main occasions in the day when everybody gets together to eat and chat . . .
>
> (Charles and Kerr 1988: 21)

Realities

The picture depicted is clear; the occasion judged important. But we need to ask about the reality of this activity. Do people ever actually eat like this, and if so, how regularly and how often? Obvious as it may seem, evidence that allows us to answer such questions is still needed before anyone can even begin to decide whether family meals are in decline. Preliminary enquiries suggest that neither sociologists nor, come to that, other types of social scientist, have paid attention to counting the frequency with which people eat with their families, round the table, at home. Unless we are all missing a major publication, there does not appear to be a single academic research study which has taken this as its central object of enquiry.[3]

Rather it seems to be the researchers in marketing or those working for mass market magazines who have collected information about mealtime patterns. For example, when *Good Housekeeping* conducted a nationwide survey of their readers in late 1993, they found that family meals were, as the magazine journalists put it, 'the daily norm' for almost half (46 per cent) of the 1,010 responses they analysed (*Good Housekeeping* 1994).[4] Or again, in June the same year, market researchers questioned some 930 adults and found that rather over half of them (57 per cent) ate with members of their household every day or almost every day, and an additional 16 per cent ate together on most days. Only 1 per cent never ate with the other people in the same house (Mintel 1993).[5] Just a couple of years later, a piece of German marketing research reported very broadly similar findings (GFM-GETAS 1995). Of the 97 per cent who reported taking dinner/supper on working days, 41 per cent said they ate 'with all other household members' and 34 per cent 'with some other household members'.[6] These three sets of information run roughly in the same direction. *Very* approximately, the family meal could be described as making a half-time appearance – but waxing or waning?

While this information is obviously to be taken seriously, there are always routine technical matters that need to be considered in determining the degree of dependability as well as generalisability of the findings. For instance, respondents in the *Good Housekeeping* survey are self-selected from its readership. Thus there is no way of knowing how far the survey is skewed in recruiting just those people who were already especially interested in the topics it covered. Nor is there any way of knowing (at least from the published material) the criteria whereby the 1,010 replies were selected for analysis from the total of 10,000 (was it really a round number?!) reported to have been received. Similarly, there is the perennial difficulty of the differences between questionnaires – the wording, ordering of questions and varying degrees of specificity.

Over and above those technicalities, we also face at least two difficulties in trying to discover whether people are eating together less often than they used to. The first is that academic researchers and market researchers are not particularly good at talking to each other – with the result that academics are generally ignorant about market researchers' findings. Even if we were all better at it, our different conditions of work make it that much harder for market researchers to make their findings available to academics than vice versa. Market research results constitute confidential, commercially sensitive material and are thus not always conventionally published in a manner generally accessible to academics or anyone else. Even when they are made more widely available, it is typically at a price way out of the reach of academics' budgets that are a tiny fraction of commercial purchasers' funds. From this follows the second difficulty. It is not easy for academics to discover whether the market researchers' findings go back as far as, for instance, the forty years referred to in the second quotation with which this chapter opened. The Taylor Nelson AGB Family Food Panel, which has been running since 1974, may contain directly relevant information, but if so it has not in any obvious way been attributably available to academics for comment or citation. If, however, market researchers' findings do not go back for the last forty years, then the question remains as to what constitutes the evidence on which that quoted observation, and others like it, was so confidently based.

Certainly some sensible guesswork is possible. Presumably, professionals in marketing would regard William Crawford's 'National Food Enquiry' (Crawford and Broadley 1938) as a piece of market research.[7] Based on interviews with approximately 5,000 families in seven major British cities between October 1936 and March 1937, the authors report that approximately half the husbands usually had their midday meal at home. They imply that the same half will be taking that meal in company with their wives and any children. Equally, though no mention is made of the matter, it is assumed that all other meals whose timing and composition are recorded, were eaten at home with the rest of the family. But the Enquiry did not, it seems, specifically ask whether families ate together.[8] So any conclusions drawn from this study about the decline of family meals, or any use of these results as some kind of baseline for the purposes of comparison, still rests on guesswork.

Real images

The chances are, then, that we have precious little evidence for the reality of family meals as an activity in which people actually do or do not engage, present or past. By contrast, an idea of family meals appears to be real enough. It does, however, have to be sought out strategically. For the idea is often evident more in somewhat shadowy form, implied, taken for granted – an image that tends, as it were, to materialise obliquely.

First – pursuing a predictable social anthropological strategy – the idea can be discovered when a threat is posed or something felt to be lacking. Consider, for example, two very disparate instances which tie together a sense of family life and round-the-table eating. In his biography of the playwright Joe Orton, John Lahr paints a portrait of the rather strange man Orton senior seems to have been. In so doing, he quotes Joe Orton's brother's comment that 'Dad was always an old man'. Lahr pursues the point:

> William never played with his children or bought them presents *or even ate dinner with the family*. He rarely went on holiday with them.
>
> (Lahr 1978: 49, emphasis added)

There is something amiss, or so Lahr seems able to presume, if a family does not share certain things, particularly meals – something unfatherly about a father who does not even eat dinner with the rest. Not eating with the family is shown to be self-evidently odd, since Lahr supposes his readers will agree, that what is ordinary about families is that they do eat together.

A parallel presumption is found in quite a different quarter. Undertaken when the post-war housing stock in Britain desperately needed restoration and overcrowding was a pressing public problem, an early 1950s study in public health and housing was almost bound to specify standards against the time when the looked-for renewal gathered speed. In the process of weighing up the pros and cons of alternative 'features of house-planning', it stipulated that a 'dining kitchen' must have sufficient 'space . . . for the family to sit comfortably round a table' (Mackintosh 1952: 158–9). There, sure enough, is the automatic assumption of the family meal, underlying the requirement for the layout, the very architectural design, as the relevant chapter title has it, for 'The family in the new house'. Repairing the breach in the ordinary way of things is the occasion for an idea, an ideal, of family life to be expressed.

The reality of the *idea* of the family meal is also noticeable when turning, equally strategically, to sources whose explicit rationale is to prescribe what family life ought to be like – such as child-rearing manuals. While there are investigations of this genre of popular literature (e.g. Hardyment 1995), a systematic analysis of their portrayal of family meals appears unavailable. A very rough-and-ready check turns up some image of the idea in nine cases out of a small, haphazard handful of eighteen twentieth-century examples. For instance:

> in the fullest sense of the word 'weaning' begins. For this process covers a great many activities and includes not only the gradual introduction of solid foods into a diet, originally entirely liquid and the introduction to spoon feeding, but also the substitution of cup drinking instead of sucking as a means of taking liquid refreshment, and finally, attendance at the family table and participation in the family meals.
>
> (Cuthbert 1948: 75)

> *From one to two years.* The baby has now reached the stage when he may have his meals with the family, sitting in his high-chair at the table with the rest.
>
> (*Good Housekeeping* Family Doctor 1955: 163, original emphasis)

This is still echoed a couple of decades later, '(o)ne year onwards, baby can now join in with most family meals' (Hull 1976) and remains evident in Penelope Leach's 1996 edition of *The Parents' A to Z.* In keeping with a later twentieth-century injunction cheerfully to accept that infants are messy on their way to learning how to wield their cutlery, manuals include advice on sensible types of bibs or the provision of an oil cloth under the chair as useful adjuncts to the child's joining everyone else at the table – but join them they are assumed likely to do.

An idea of family meals, however real, remains just that, an idea. It is thus potentially redolent of ideology, social prescription and ideals. The idea portrayed is real enough, but that is not to say it is a faithful reproduction of some truth in the way that a photograph is (erroneously) supposed to be. Furthermore, there is no way of being sure that those who speak approvingly of family meals are consciously, deliberately even, perpetuating only a favourable version. A more discomfiting reality is, of course, also on record.[9]

Only a couple of examples (once again coming from disparate quarters) are needed, recollecting grimmer sides to family eating.[10] Burgoyne and Clark's study of second marriages provides a further instance. One of their informants complained of her husband's lack of understanding in his dealings with Jonathan (aged 4) yet simultaneously felt guilty about contradicting her husband in front of the child:

> When our Jonathan's poorly . . . he's mardy, *very* mardy. . . . This last fortnight . . . he goes off food altogether when he's poorly, he'll drink a tap dry . . . but he plays wi' his food then and Martin gets rather angry wi' him . . . like at t'dinner table t'other day, I forget what it were we had to eat . . . but instead of telling his Dad that he didn't want it, he were moaning so. . . . Martin shouted at him and the tears come and then I said 'Well you shouldn't have done that, he's not very well and you know he's poorly' and . . . when I thought about it after . . . I should have held me tongue and waited while our Jonathan had gone out and then told him.
>
> (Burgoyne and Clark 1984: 170–1)

The second comes from another biography, that of Raymond Postgate, the founder of *The Good Food Guide*, written by his elder son and daughter-in-law. It describes the relationship between Raymond Postgate and his wife:

> Ray's marriage . . . had settled down to a new level of affection and understanding, though they knew each other's faults well and Daisy, especially, rarely hesitated to speak of them. They had a tendency to bicker: they would engage in ritual arguments and criticisms, each knowing perfectly well how the other would react, even to the words, but both seemingly compelled to keep the ritual going. They forbore to some extent in company, but the children were part of the furniture in this regard. *Meal times were preferred bickering times*; the boys usually remained tuned out, but could sometimes shame them to stop by speaking each one's part for them.
>
> (Postgate and Postgate 1994: 185)

We are left, nevertheless, with snatches of evidence that the family meal continues to be an ideal towards which people should strive, an aspiration that may be powerfully expressed. Charles and Kerr's reports of younger English women's stress on the importance of families eating together was noted earlier in this chapter. Similar aspirations are reported for some American parents in full-time employment who 'feel frustrated and defeated' when their commitments limit their arranging family meals of the sort they remember:

> good meals on the table. It was more of a family thing. You know, my dad got home at a certain time, and we always ate dinner after he got home. . . . Now it's like a helter skelter routine.

> you have a real discussion at the dinner table, like we used to when I was a kid, you can give a person a chance to let you in on their life. What they were doing all day when they weren't with you.
>
> (DeVault 1991: 52–3)

Much the same aspirations are reported from small-scale studies in Sweden. Anxious lest the family meal is indeed disappearing, Sören Jansson's study of both middle- and working-class people in Stockholm shows they go to considerable lengths to avoid eating alone (Jansson 1988) – findings that were later fully confirmed (Wall 1995). Frihammar's (1995) work, though, reveals a difference. These findings represent a refinement, and suggest that upper middle-class women place heavy emphasis on the family meal as vital to being a family. This is in complete contrast to working-class women who still value the family, but accord the meal comparatively little significance as a symbol of it (Frihammar 1995).[11] And in a study still in progress, Rosemary Kyle finds a persistent allegiance to the family meal amongst middle-aged professional men in the South of England.[12]

> We try hard at the weekends to have at least one meal together as a family.

> I much like the idea of sitting down with the family in the evening and having a meal together, though sometimes it's not always possible because of people's commitments . . . inevitably you can't all dovetail together.

At the same time, the second informant recalled 'horrendous' childhood memories of family meals, especially those with his grandparents: strictness, formal table manners, an 'intimidating atmosphere', while another of Kyle's informants stressed that:

> we make a point of eating together as a family . . . at least three of us sit down together every evening except Monday. It is an important time of day, especially when the kids were younger. I do think it's important to sit down together at a table – yes, we sit at the table – it's a large dining table and I sit opposite my wife and [son] sits opposite [daughter] and at the end of the table.

The snatches of material about the idea of the family meal as an aspiration seem much more commonly to reflect an image of an ideal at which everyone should be aiming. More rarely – and thus perhaps more tellingly – quite the opposite aspiration can also be detected. Even if family meals are not the occasion for bickering, but come closer to a pleasant if lively image of sociability, not everyone wants to stick with them. A salutary finding appears in Barbara Dobson and her colleagues' (1994) recent study of forty-eight low-income families, all, it must be added, with dependent children.[13] Most of them ate together in the evenings. Some did so because they considered it important and gave them the chance to talk; others did so, however, simply because it was cheaper. A quarter resented the fact that they had to eat together in order to economise by avoiding cooking a second meal or not having to keep food hot.

> We'd sit down and eat in the evenings together but sometimes I get fed up of eating with the kids and I'd love to have my dinner just with [her husband] later in the evening but the kids can't wait. They're hungry when they come in from school and it's all I can get them to do to wait until tea time. (New income support recipient, couple, more than one child)

> We always eat with the children and have done for a long time but it'd be nice not having to. That's what you notice living on benefit, you'd think, well he's not working so he's got loads of time for himself, but it's not like that at all. You can't afford to go out so you stay in, I mean, don't get me wrong, I love my kids, but they're kids and sometimes at tea I'm more a referee than anything else. It'd be nice to let them eat on their own sometimes and let them get on with it. (Long-term unemployed, husband, couple, more than one child)

> (Dobson *et al.* 1994: 18)

That woman's wish for a break from tea-time peace-keeping may well evoke some sympathy. However, if we are to take seriously claims that family meals are declining, then the search for evidence to support them will need, at a minimum, to separate reports of frequency from articulations of an idealised image. The latter may be real enough, but they concern the reality of an idea that may not represent actual activities so much as images of family living to which people aspire. Furthermore we have to cater for the possibility that the relation between actuality and aspiration is liable to be inverse. Obviously, those who consider their family does not eat together often enough are likely to be making this judgement against an aspiration which has a positive image of mealtimes – *and* vice versa.

HISTORY, MYTH AND GOLDEN AGES

At this point, the discussion shifts focus to take a closer look at two questions posed at the beginning: what kind of family, what kind of worry? So far, this chapter has uncritically accepted the cornflake packet picture of the family, and with it, perpetuated the all too common elision between family and household. Yet, the two need to be distinguished for analytic purposes: self-evidently those who live in the same dwelling, the domestic group, need not be related by either blood or marriage.

Family, household – and history

Family forms and household structures have varied very consider-ably in different socio-economic circumstances or social classes. Indeed, households do not necessarily constitute the boundary of ordinary family life. Having a meal with certain members of the family means, by definition, not having it with others. In their classic investigation of family life of South Wales in the late 1950s and early 1960s, Rosser and Harris noticed that it was common for married sons regularly to call at their mothers' homes for meals:

'George comes in here *every* morning at a quarter past eight for breakfast on his way to work', says Mrs Barry, aged 63, of Little Gam Street near the Town Centre. 'He lives out on the Portmead Estate and works in a gents' outfitters in the Kingsway near here. He doesn't start till nine, but his wife has

to get to her job at the Trading Estate in Fforestfach by eight. And *of course* I get his dinner for him here *every* day too.'
(Rosser and Harris 1965: 153, emphasis added)

Even where household and family coincide, internal social divisions are evident, not least at meals. Littlejohn's remarkable, and insufficiently well-known, study of life in a rural parish in the Scottish Borders, reports contrasts between working- and middle-class family meals:

The higher position of the wife in the middle-class household vis-à-vis the husband is expressed in the ceremony surrounding meals, particularly tea, a meal at which all members of the family in all classes are usually present. There is a marked difference between the working class on the one hand and the middle classes on the other in the way behaviour is patterned during the meals, a difference which aptly expresses the difference in status of the wife in the two sorts of household.
(Littlejohn 1963: 127)

As he shows, the working-class wife is more like a servant or a waitress at a meal than a fellow diner.[14]

It is often forgotten that, over the last 150–200 years the children of upper-class, wealthy and aristocratic families *never* ate with the rest of the family. Indeed their whole childhood could be passed in an almost wholly self-contained life in the nursery over which Nanny presided (and for the boys, later, at boarding school, the girls with a governess or schoolmistress at home). They might only see their parents, most likely their mother, once a day for, say, half an hour.[15] The food they ate was quite different from that of the adults. Children's menus were typically of bland, monotonous foods, with a limited variety of dishes, utterly unlike the elaborate meals placed before their parents (Gathorne-Hardy 1972).[16] Here the household consisted of all members of a nuclear family – together with living-in servants – but age put kin members at separate dinner tables, as did social class (servants ate separately too).

Over the same century and a half there is the other end of the scale of advantage. Amongst this stratum there must have been large numbers of exceptionally poor families whose overcrowded, bleak homes never even acquired a table. Certainly, we have reports of such severe poverty in the last century and well into this, that women were led to go without food altogether so that their husbands (the breadwinners) and the children could eat (Pember Reeves 1913, Spring Rice 1939, and see data for the poor in the 1970s summarised in Graham 1984). In these circumstances, the notion of a sociable family meal is likely to be somewhat wide of the mark. Even if everyone did have something to eat, husbands were still accorded better, more interesting or higher-status food. Ross (1994) reports this for Londoners in the late 1800s (see Delphy 1979 for nineteenth-century rural France) and Charles and Kerr (1988) found the same in the North-East of England in the 1980s amongst averagely well-off households. In these instances, household and nuclear family coincide and its members may well forgather to eat at the same time. Access to the food available is, however, gendered – which, like the gendering in Littlejohn's study, raises a query about the 'togetherness' assumed in a notion of family meals.

Gender, age and class all, then, start to break up an image of sharing at the dinner table by reflecting internal divisions of status and power in the domestic group. It would, then, seem reasonable to suppose that the idea of the family commentators have in mind when worrying about the decline of their shared meal, is probably an ideal-typical model of the middle-class and (respectable) working-class family. This gives rise to the speculation that those who are most likely to express anxiety about the possible disappearance of families eating together are those whose own social origins are the source of an allegiance to middle-class values, and the middle-class valuation of family meals. But, of course, further investigation is needed to be sure.

Myth – and history

It was noted at the beginning of this chapter that amongst those accepting that the family meal is a thing of the past were sociologists, including recently, Pasi Falk. He places the dissolution, the 'marginalisation' of the shared meal at the centre of his vision of what he calls the 'modern eating-culture' (Falk 1994: 29). Unlike the 'non-ritual eating of tribal societies', Falk argues that what is new to the modern condition is the 'decline of the ritual meal and . . . the rise of the food industry' (Falk 1994: 30). The (only) source Falk provides in support of the veracity of his reference to this modern novelty is Harvey Levenstein's (1988) social history of the revolution in American eating. And, in turn, a key source Levenstein provides is the classic of American community studies, Robert Lynd and Helen Lynd's *Middletown*, alias Muncie, a town of some 30,000 population in Indiana.

Their study was published in 1929. In the present context, that date is rather important, and leads this discussion back to the very first quotation with which this chapter opened. For it is from *Middletown* that the quotation comes (Lynd and Lynd 1929: 153–4). And the data which showed a 'conscious effort to "save meal-times . . . for the family"' were collected between January 1924 and June 1925, a fraction over seventy years ago. This places the previous generation's family reunions at the dinner table, to which the Lynds refer, in the final decade of the *nineteenth* century. As much to the point, it dates the existence of an established anxiety about the decline of the family meal, in at least one small American town, not so long after the end of the First World War.

The other two quotations at the beginning of this chapter may differ somewhat in vocabulary or style, but arguably, they purport to record the same change in eating arrangements and express the same concern as the Lynds reported for the USA. Both, though, are British; the source of the second is a booklet written by Tim Lang and colleagues (Lang 1989), while the third, published even more recently in a medical journal, is from a 'think piece' by John Davis, Emeritus Professor of Paediatrics (Davis 1995).[17]

At this point, two alternative possibilities have seriously to be considered. One is that even if firm and detailed evidence over a good number of decades is lacking, the Lynds' data might suggest that reports of the fairly long-standing decline of the family meal are well founded. There are, however, a couple of difficulties with this possibility. Though the fact that the Lynds returned to Muncie ten years later to conduct a re-study holds out the promise of providing us with some trend data, their attention was repeatedly turned on to enquiring about the effects of the Depression. It is striking that their discussion of eating in *Middletown in Transition* is far less about meals and much more about food – its cost and whether children were getting enough (Lynd and Lynd 1937). They make no mention of mealtimes as family reunions, although they do note that remarkably little of life generally had changed since their first study. Second, though the material is slender, the frequency of shared meals reported in *Middletown* does not sound that much different from far more recent reports. The decline, then, would not seem to be proceeding steadily since the inter-war years but to have already occurred, with frequency of shared meals remaining depressed ever since.

As plausible – or just possibly more so – is quite a different interpretation. This alternative proposes that an anxiety lest the family meal is waning is also to be understood as if it were a standing item on the agenda of twentieth-century public commentary on the nature of family life. It is exactly parallel to Pimlott's observation that it is 'part of the tradition that Christmas is never as it used to be' (Pimlott 1978: 179). In this view, one generation reflects on life the generation before, not only finds it altered, but judges it wanting. Each successive generation does exactly the same. Thus it is a constant that the past is mourned, the golden age feared lost.

The second interpretation has to stand until there is sound argument and good evidence to discard it. Until that time, 'family meals as a thing of the past' must continue to be followed by a question mark. Not only do we probably have insufficient evidence either way, but we also may be looking for quite the wrong type of evidence, confusing historical fact with the necessary myths which human beings create to help make collective sense of the social arrangements they inherit and the social changes they experience. There is, then, a good deal more steady investigation to be undertaken before any conclusion about family meals can be confidently and intelligently drawn.

NOTES

This chapter is a revised version of a paper with the same title, presented at the 1995 Annual Meeting of the British Association for the Advancement of Science, Anthropology Section, and is addressed as much to colleagues beyond the academic community as those within it. I wish to thank Pat Caplan, who was the 1995 Section President for the invitation to speak on that occasion and for her benign and helpful editorial hand; also Madeleine Gantley, Hilary Rose, Laura McKenzie, Taylor Nelson plc, and, in particular, Paula McDonnell, Paula McGrath and Jane Worsley of the BBC Radio 4 Science Unit. I should like to record my appreciation of Phil Strong's comments during the early stages of preparing this paper together with his suggestions for illustrations; he died before it could be finished.

1 See e.g. features in *The Independent*, 19 December 1994, 'Death of the British Sunday', and 14 June 1995 on childhood. Also, Hopkins's popular social history in which he comments:

In the intimate history of most British families in the Fifties the Day the Television Came forms a sort of postwar watershed. . . . The sacrosanct ritual of meals was broken. Gathered before the hypnotic screen on the low 'television chairs' that now made their appearance in the shops, families took their food from large 'television plates', gropingly in the half-darkness.

(Hopkins 1963: 331)

2 It is as pertinent to ask: 'What kind of meal?' – but that will have to wait for another occasion.

3 There are, of course, studies which do deal with the topic in some fashion or another perhaps introduced by respondents, or mentioned in passing as an adjunct to debating other topics. Some are drawn on later in this chapter. Some are constituent projects in the Economic and Social Research Council (UK) Research Programme 'The Nation's Diet: The Social Science of Food Choice' of which the present author is Director. None, though, concentrate wholly or fully on the topic.

4 Some regional variation is recorded: 'families in the Midlands and East Anglia are most likely to eat together daily (51 per cent), but only 42 per cent of their counterparts in London and the South-East do so.'

5 This work also reports regional variation with respondents in Scotland and the North-West most likely to say they eat together daily (70 per cent and 62 per cent respectively), London (53 per cent) and Yorkshire/North-East (52 per cent) least.

6 Covering both the West and the East, 1,250 people over the age of 14 were interviewed during September 1995.

7 See his own *Personal Introduction* to the book.

8 Or if it did, for some reason the authors decided against including the findings in the report.

9 The more favourable version was taken up and given a rosy polish by advertisers in the UK with a long-running series of television commercials for a stock cube (Vincenzi 1985).

10 *The Intelligent Parents' Manual* is one of the few that discusses children's presence at the meal table at some length, spelling out pros and cons, proposing solutions to difficulties – one of which is to have a young child eat separately during the week. The authors nonetheless observe that '(i)n most cases . . . parents will feel that generally the whole family should take their meals together, and that a child should feed alone only exceptionally' (Powdermaker and Grimes 1953: 114–15).

11 I am grateful to Sören Jansson for summarising his own, Wall's and Frihammar's findings in English for me.

12 I am grateful to Rosemary Kyle for permission to refer to, and quote from her work in progress.

13 Half the families were lone parents, the other half couples, with the majority of the children under 7 years old.

14 Littlejohn's exposition of the 'tea ceremony' stands as an object lesson of the detailed observation that ought to be undertaken by

those of us attempting to develop adequate understandings of the complex social phenomena eating occasions represent.

15 Churchill wrote of his mother that: 'I loved her dearly – but at a distance.' And talking about food Bernard Shaw wrote:

> I hated the servants and liked my mother because on the one or two rare and delightful occasions when she buttered my bread for me, she buttered it thickly instead of merely wiping a knife on it. Her almost complete neglect of me had the advantage that I could idolise her to the utmost pitch of my imagination. . . . It was a privilege to be taken for a walk or a visit with her, or on an excursion.
>
> (Gathorne-Hardy 1972: 78)

16 Boiled meat, steamed fish, cabbage and milk-based puddings – rice and tapioca – appeared in the nursery. Strictness in routine extended to meals, menus and finishing everything on the plate – any food that was left uneaten was liable to reappear at the next meal, even the one after that.

17 Though flattering, it is mildly curious that Davis's one item of bibliography is my own edited collection (Murcott 1983) which, as far as I am aware, can claim to support nothing in his article, except the broadest possible generality. And, by coincidence, Davis gives his article the identical title to the present chapter – minus the question mark.

REFERENCES

Burgoyne, J. and Clark, D. (1984) *Making a Go of It*, London: Routledge and Kegan Paul.

Charles, N. and Kerr, M. (1988) *Women, Food and Families*, Manchester: Manchester University Press.

Crawford, W. and Broadley, H. (1938) *The People's Food*, London: William Heinemann.

Cuthbert, A. (1948) *Housewife Baby Book*, London: Hulton Press.

Davis, J.A. (1995) 'Family meals: a thing of the past', *Archives of Disease in Childhood* 73: 356.

Delphy, C. (1979) 'Sharing the same table', in C. Harris (ed.) *The Sociology of the Family*, Sociological Review Monograph 28, Keele: Keele University Press.

DeVault, M.L. (1991) *Feeding the Family*, Chicago: Chicago University Press.

Dobson, B., Beardsworth, A., Keil, T. and Walker, R. (1994) *Diet, Choice and Poverty*, London: Family Policy Studies Centre.

Falk, P. (1994) *The Consuming Body*, London: Sage.

Fischler, C. (1979) 'Gastro-nomie et gastro-anomie', *Communications* 31: 189–210.

Frihammar, M. (1995) *Dinner and Class*, Stockholm: Institutet för Folklivsforskning.

Gathorne-Hardy, J. (1972) *The Rise and Fall of the British Nanny*, London: Arrow Books.

GFM-GETAS (Gesellschaft fur Marketing-, Kommunikations- und Sozialforschung mbH) (1995) *Meals in Germany*, Hamburg: GFM-GETAS.

Good Housekeeping (1994) 'Women prefer a good meal to sex', Press Release, 31 January, London: The National Magazine Company Ltd.

Good Housekeeping Family Doctor (1955) *Baby Book*, London: The National Magazine Company Ltd.

Graham, H. (1984) *Women, Health and the Family*, Brighton, Sussex: Harvester.

Hardyment, C. (1995) *Perfect Parents*, Oxford: Oxford University Press.

Hopkins, H. (1963) *The New Look*, London: Secker and Warburg.

Hull, S. (1976) *Cooking for a Baby*, Harmondsworth: Penguin.

Jansson, S. (1988) 'Maten och myterna' (Food and myths), *Vår Föda* 40, Suppl. 2: 44–203.

Lahr, J. (1978) *Prick up your Ears*, Harmondsworth: Penguin.

Lang, T., Dib, S., Cole-Hamilton, I. and Lobstein, T. (1989) *This Food Business*, London: New Statesman and Society.

Leach, P. (1996) *The Parents' A to Z*, Harmondsworth: Penguin.

Levenstein, H. (1988) *Revolution at the Table*, New York: Oxford University Press.

Littlejohn, J. (1963) *Westrigg*, London: Routledge and Kegan Paul.

Lynd, R.S. and Lynd, H.M. (1929) *Middletown*, London: Constable.

—— (1937) *Middletown in Transition*, London: Constable.

Mackintosh, J.M. (1952) *Housing and Family Life*, London: Cassell.

Mintel (1993) 'Cooking and eating habits', *Leisure Intelligence* 4: 1–14.

Mintz, S.W. (1985) *Sweetness and Power*, New York: Viking.

Murcott, A. (1983) *The Sociology of Food and Eating*, Aldershot: Gower.

Pember Reeves, M. (1913) *Round About a Pound a Week*, London: Virago.

Pimlott, J.A.R. (1978) *The Englishman's Christmas*, Hassocks, Sussex: Harvester.

Postgate, J. and Postgate, M. (1994) *A Stomach for Dissent*, Keele: Keele University Press.

Powdermaker, F. and Grimes, L. (1953) *The Intelligent Parents' Manual*, 2nd edn, Harmondsworth: Penguin.

Ross, E. (1994) *Love and Toil: Motherhood in Outcast London, 1870–1918*, Oxford: Oxford University Press.

Rosser, C. and Harris, C. (1965) *The Family and Social Change*, London: Routledge and Kegan Paul.

Spring Rice, M. (1939) *Working-Class Wives*, Harmondsworth: Penguin.

Vincenzi, P. (1985) *Taking Stock*, London: Collins.

Wall, M. (1995) *Den gemensamma måltiden* (The shared meal), Stockholm: Institutet för Folklivsforskning.

Chapter 3

Marriages, weddings and their cakes

Simon Charsley

In the classic British wedding cake, form triumphantly replaces any consideration of eatability, let alone of nutrition. Its cutting rather than its eating is the focus of attention. Categorically it belongs with foods but it highlights their capacity to carry huge loads of social and cultural significance, almost to the point of caricature.

As a spin-off from a study of rites of marrying in Glasgow in the 1980s (Charsley 1991),[1] the intricate history of this amazing creation was researched and an account of it eventually published in 1992 as *Wedding Cakes and Cultural History*.[2] Though stirrings of change were already clear at the period, and are discussed there, it was the classic form of the British wedding cake which demanded attention. This was an essentially mysterious object, constructed to an elaborate prescription but provided with little of what the anthropologist away from home might have termed 'native exegesis'. Though always thought of as a cake, in the singular, it was, ideally and frequently in practice, a construction of three cakes of declining size set one above the other. The two upper 'tiers' were raised on sets of pillars, each standing on the top surface of the tier below. Each was iced and decorated in a distinctive style of piped 'royal' icing, generally white; each was a reduced reproduction of the one below. Inside the shell of hard white icing was a fruit cake, heavy, dark and spiced. Hardly anyone, either the makers or those who might spend the equivalent of a week's salary on such a cake for their wedding, had anything to say in explanation of the form or its meanings.

This became the lead problem for the research: what part had meanings played, despite contemporary unawareness of them, in the creation and continuation of a food item which had so

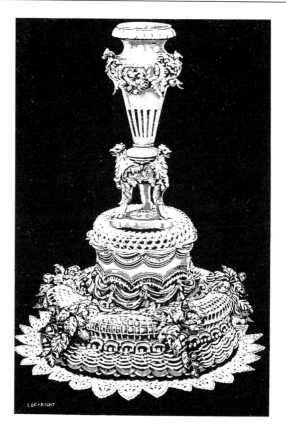

Figure 1 A scraper-board picture of a cake by Herr T. Willy, published in his *All About Piping* (1891, London)

transcended its origins that its major use was to be symbolically cut? An essential element of the wedding it certainly was, but it was not uncommon for those marrying to announce that they did not actually like it. This mattered little, since eating was not part of the prescription, a voluntary extra only. The attempt was made to trace the interplay of meanings with other factors, primarily commercial opportunity and the initiatives of the trade. As befitted a creation in a commercial society, the wedding cake was revealed as essentially motivated and formed by commerce, though commerce had had to work within constraints of available meaning and practice in doing so.

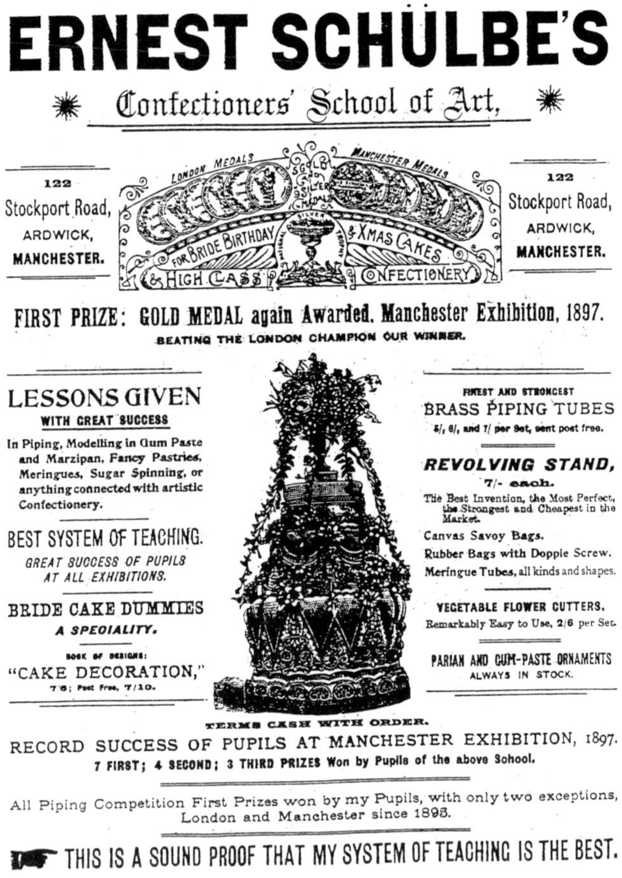

Figure 2 An advertisement for E. Schülbé, from *The British Baker* (1897)

The form achieved in the early twentieth century enjoyed a remarkable stability throughout most of the remainder of it. The paucity both of substantial change and of attributions of meaning was the twentieth-century phenomenon. It was argued that this combination of stability and lack of interpretation was not accidental: the cake had become simply an aspect of the culturally defined way in which marriages were made. Meanings for objects and practices, it seemed on the basis of this evidence, are very variably pursued, except by the intruding anthropologist for whom

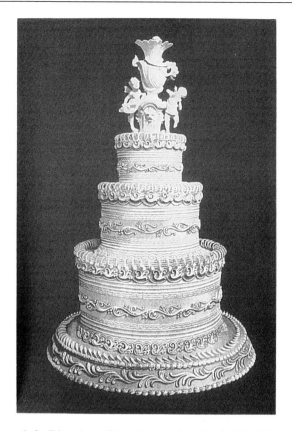

Figure 3 A slide taken of the picture of a cake by Mr F. Pass of Glasgow, 1st Prize winner in the Scottish section of the London International Exhibition, 1902. Reprinted from T. P. Lewis & A. G. Bromley, *The Book of Cakes* (1903, London: Maclaren)

everything is, or should be, a puzzle needing explanation. Only if and to the extent that interpretation began were the accepted form and procedures in danger. In the 1980s, feminist concerns about the gender inequality which marriage customs might be signifying did occasionally provide the impetus to such interpretation and thereby a threat to the cake's place in proceedings. Only when, exceptionally, those with power to change things start identifying meanings does interpretation come into dynamic relationship with custom, either sustaining existing practice or challenging it. If a single wedding ring or the cutting of the wedding cake are

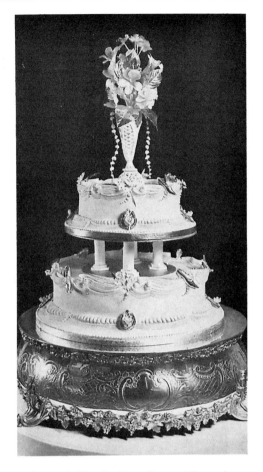

Figure 4 Classical two-tier wedding cake.
Reprinted with kind permission of Fortnum and Mason, from their
brochure of Wedding and Celebration Cakes (1968, London)

attributed meanings which, for example, offend gender sensibilities, then such practices may begin to change.

As had, however, already become clear even in the period between the beginning of the research and the writing of the book, an era was ending. The prescription was changing. From the perspective of the later 1990s it comes to seem that it is no longer stability but a radical collapse of the old which demands the explanation. What can be seen more clearly now is the dynamic

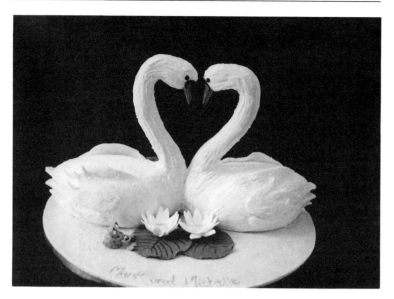

Figure 5 Photograph of Swans Cake (1996, London).
Reprinted by kind permission of Jane Asher Party Cakes

relationship between cakes and their weddings, not only between the new wedding cake and contemporary marriage but also between Victorian marriage and the cake which was created for its making.

COMMERCE AND THE CREATION OF THE WEDDING CAKE

In 1763 Elizabeth Raffald, the housekeeper in an aristocratic household in Cheshire, married the head gardener, moved to Manchester and set up a confectioner's shop in Market Place. Her husband went into business as a seedsman. She was an energetic lady and her enterprises quickly multiplied, amongst them the publication in 1769 of one of the great recipe books of the century, *The Experienced English Housekeeper.* This is a remarkable compilation, with 'near 800 original receipts', but its relevance is that it contained instructions 'To make a Bride Cake' and for its icing. In the context of her shopkeeping this is likely to have been an explicit exercise in product differentiation: a rich fruit cake, original in including a large quantity of candied citrus fruits arranged in layers, was labelled 'bride cake'. It was then further differentiated in its icing. Here she instructed her readers first to put on a layer of almond icing and then to cover this with a layer of ordinary white icing (Raffald 1769: 242–4). This was not only the first published recipe for a cake specifically for weddings, it was also the first appearance of what was to become a classic British combination of icings. There is good circumstantial evidence that Mrs Raffald had invented it as a design for selling in her confectioner's shop.[3] Her book went through some thirty-six editions up to 1825. Well before that, but after her death in 1781, others were publishing versions of her scheme too.

Mrs Raffald provides a pragmatic starting point for a process which did not in reality have one. It was the nearest the wedding cake came to being an invention rather than a gradual construction. Though her contribution was important, it represents a moment only in the building together of a series of elements which were themselves products of experimentation over a period of centuries. The oldest was some kind of bread or cake appearing in marriage festivities; then it was the use of a rich, spiced, dried-fruit mixture; then that it should be iced, eventually using Elizabeth Raffald's double-icing; then that cakes of declining size should be piled up and combined into a single cake; then that its decoration should be icing piped in a characteristic style to which we shall return; finally that the tiers should be separated by pillars and should match.

To list in this way the main elements of the product finally achieved is, however, misleading. It hides the open-ended creativity of the process, ignoring alternative possibilities and innovations which were tried but failed. Mrs Raffald's own layering of 'sweetmeats' was never widely followed and her double icing took until the middle of the nineteenth century to become a fixed feature of the developing wedding cake and thence of Christmas and other new celebration cakes as they were created.

In the course of the progression however, cake as something appropriate for display and eating at weddings became *the* wedding cake, just one for each wedding and a prime focus for it. The mixture used up to the present is the direct descendant of the first kind of British 'cake' as that term is now understood. This was the product of experimental enriching of breads from the sixteenth to the early eighteenth centuries. A separate tradition of monumental sugar work introduced the high-rising cake, particularly in the context of the series of Victorian royal weddings through the latter half of the century. It was not until late in the century that the shape of royal cakes began to be taken up for the commercial product by piling cakes of declining size one on another. Piped white 'royal' icing became its standard form of decoration. At the beginning of the twentieth century, this commercial cake itself achieved a distinctively architectural appearance by raising the tiers on pillars. Looked at retrospectively it can be seen that each new successful development was locked into place by subsequent developments. Once pillars separated the tiers, a style of decoration treating each tier as a miniature of the one below it helped fix the separation of tiers.

This was the Edwardian form, the classic British wedding cake which was to last through most of the rest of the century. However debased and mechanical its decoration might become – as indeed it often did – it had achieved an unmistakable form which could be reproduced endlessly in different sizes and qualities to suit circumstances and the varying depth of pockets. It was to be widely copied around the world, together with the white wedding dress, as a characteristic wedding symbol in the hegemonic Anglo-American cultural array.

Throughout most of the cake's history, experimentation and popularisation were the work of the bakery and confectionery trades. Few amateurs ever had the skills or the confidence to match the 'professional' and ever more elaborate standards set by the trade. For Queen Victoria's own wedding in 1840, and increasingly for the series of her children's weddings starting in 1858, leading firms supplied cakes of monumental size and form, exciting widespread interest and publicity. To start with, these cakes were additional to the official cakes, generally prepared in-house by royal confectioners, but the trade gradually took over. A series of exhibitions also encouraged competition at levels of cost and ambition well beyond commercial practicality. Wedding cakes featured at events in the 1880s but it was a series of annual baking and confectionery exhibitions held in London from 1893 and in Manchester from a few years later that gave them and their makers the ultimate incentive for originality and the achievement of the highest standards. Stars, most notably Ernest Schülbé of Manchester, had a platform on which to display themselves and their newly fashionable art of piping, to be applied first and foremost to these impractical specimens. The distinction between what was required for a 'five-guinea cake' for the London exhibitions, which would have taken months to produce and was only to be looked at, and real cakes which could be made and sold for so much per pound, was not missed by commentators (e.g. Gommez 1899: 11–13). Schülbé, Herr Willy – always so named – and Gommez were the leading proponents, exploiting an air of Continental sophistication for the development of what was in fact a distinctively British enthusiasm. They all had schools of piping and confectionery in the 1890s, directing their efforts primarily to the trade. They wrote instructional books and developed and stocked equipment that baker-confectioners would need if they were to move into the field. Before piping skills had spread widely, ready-piped tops and even shells to cover a whole cake could be purchased by inexperienced bakers. Piping was the key: for a time ordinary bakers, even those with sufficient high-class trade to have a market for such expensive goods, were left behind as the expert and ambitious fired increasingly widespread enthusiasm with their amazing designs and strong publicity. In time however, with training, the ordinary artisan was going to be able to produce cakes decorated in the distinctive style which the leaders developed, flowing yet petrified. They would do it with a polish and neatness not easily copied by the amateur, and they would do it with impressive speed, making commercial production practicable and profitable.

The wedding cake as it developed was therefore essentially a design for producing and selling.[4] Marchant, a learned trade propagandist whose small book was circulated by one of the leading London firms with their price list in 1879, was essentially right when he wrote that bakers had 'invented and still manufacture the Wedding Cake'. 'The composition of the plum pudding is essentially a domestic duty', he declared, but the cake 'is a work of art and necessitates the employment of diverse talents of the highest order' (Marchant 1879: 80). It was not, that is to say, a folk object taken up by commerce. When cakes of the classic form were produced by people for their own use, they were attempting to copy what commerce had already created.

MEANINGFUL CHARACTERISTICS OF THE CLASSIC WEDDING CAKE

Aspects of the classic cake as it developed related to a range of considerations and factors, to royal influences, to what was happening to culinary display in the Victorian period, as well as to the development of the baking and confectionery trades and in particular their vigorous experimentation in the 1890s. But key features were directly meaningful in relation to marriage. These were in part readable at the time, even if few attempted it; in part they have become clearer with subsequent change. A number of features developed, that is to say, not through any intentional significance built into them, though this could be attempted, but because they were part of patterns of wider scope developing at the period.

The first aspect to note is the development of the unique relationship between a cake and a wedding. The contrast between the usual older term, 'bridecake', and 'wedding cake' which gradually replaced it is relevant here. 'Bride-' was once the designation for almost everything to do with a wedding though now it survives only precariously as the last relic of this form, 'bridegroom', is reduced to simple 'groom'. 'Bridecake' was originally cake or cakes of any kind associated with a wedding. There was nothing fixed about the number of such cakes. As 'cake' was first elaborated and became more costly and then was taken up by the ever-growing Victorian middle class, mainly less wealthy than their predecessors from the gentry and aristocracy, a definitely singular 'wedding cake' took over, a single object strongly identified with a particular event.

Royal cakes highlight the significance of this change. They continued to be multiple even when uniqueness had become established for others, but they were of two increasingly divergent kinds. The official cakes represented the wider significance of the union, in particular the alliance between the countries and/or families involved. Cakes as distributable and portable containers of meaning carried the message of the wedding, indeed participation in it, to significant others whether they were physically present or not, and cake for this purpose continued to be produced in the quantities required. The other kind of royal cake, the private, in contrast stood chiefly for the personal aspect of the marriage, the union of two individuals in terms of an institution which was definitionally the same for them as for anyone else. Private royal cakes accordingly followed, if very grandly, the evolving patterns in the population generally, for most of whom it was the personal aspect which loomed largest. In terms of their cakes, as in other ways, royalty were both the same and different.

Forms of decoration are revealing too. A clear intention in the decoration of official cakes was to identify the couple marrying and what they stood for. There would be coats of arms and emblems and often even Wedgwood-style cameo portraits of the couple. Though the trade sometimes tried to extend this style of decoration to other cakes, it was only taken up in relation to aristocratic marriages for which the model of the royal alliance was closely relevant. Banners were the one exception. Originated in a royal context, their use spread in the late nineteenth century and persisted in some corners of Scotland into the mid-twentieth. They typically showed the initials of the parties, originally embroidered on pieces of silk suspended banner-like from miniature poles stuck into the cake. Apart from these, what seemed relevant for ordinary weddings was, as can now be recognised, a determinedly anonymous style. Piping is well-suited for writing – names and greetings have always been prominent motifs for other kinds of occasion – but for the wedding cake any kind of writing, with the one very limited exception already mentioned, was always firmly rejected. It was not, as far as can be seen, that a decision was ever taken; writing was simply understood as inappropriate for such cakes. Piping turned out also to be ideally suited to producing an elaborate, repetitive but non-representational style of decoration, and it was for this that it was adopted with such enthusiasm as the basic decorative technique. Any further decoration took conspicuously limited and stereotyped forms, depending heavily on flowers and foliage, either natural or artificial or simply providing motifs. Two others, long established before the classic cake developed, were turtle doves, proverbial for their 'conjugal affection and constancy' as *The Oxford English Dictionary* puts it, and Cupids, baby male figures of the son of Venus and Mercury, the personification of love. Such ornaments were probably never entirely eliminated but they tended to be squeezed out by the elaborated piped designs as these developed towards the end of the century. Even in the twentieth, when the older forms returned and were supplemented by others, decorations remained conspicuously limited and stereotyped in the forms used, relating in highly conventional ways to the fact of wedding but avoiding any individualised reference to the parties themselves.

Colour is a third significant characteristic, after uniqueness and decorative anonymity. The ideal of whiteness was part of the definition of icing as that oddly named substance was originally evolved. At the beginning, therefore, if cakes were to be iced, there was no choice of colour: they were bound to be more or less white. The association of white with purity is ancient, and, as icing developed, achieving the purest white possible was an unquestioned goal. The better the quality of the sugar used, the whiter the product would be. Whiter therefore meant higher quality and greater expense. In the late eighteenth century however, as part of a differentiation of kinds and shapes of cake, colouring for icing excited attention. Edinburgh appears to have been a notable source for this development. There the great architectural scheme of the New Town was maturing and society was exceptional in its liveliness and brilliance (Youngson 1966: 235ff.). As the arts of living flourished, confectionery had its part to play and in the first decade of the nineteenth century the confectioners of Edinburgh took up the colouring and decoration of cakes with particular enthusiasm. Some of the earliest accounts come from cookery books published in the city (Frazer 1806, Caird 1809), but cakes for weddings were not at first included. The bride's pie was still the Scottish speciality at the time, and it probably inhibited the use of English-style cakes. Subsequently they do appear however, but whereas in London allegiance to the traditional white icing was retained, in Edinburgh it was then decided that they should be pink. Colour was, that is to say, made an explicitly meaningful difference. With the pink icing went a wider and more romantic vocabulary of ornament than any yet noted from the South. There were not only Cupids and turtle doves but 'torches, flames, darts and other emblematic devices of this kind' (Dods 1833: 321–2, 369).

It was the southern definition however which won out throughout Britain and the reason, there can be little doubt, was the power of an idea. When decoration for the wedding cake began in the South, it did so in the context of another major celebration cake already established there, the Twelfth cake, baked for the celebration at the end of the Christmas season. That was coloured and decorated with representational forms, often toy-like in their inspiration (Henisch 1984). The wedding cake contrasted conspicuously with this formula. It was to remain white-iced, restrained and serious in its decoration. Flowers and foliage were, as has been noted, the chief item or inspiration. If colour were to be used at all, it would be introduced sparingly through flowers. It can hardly have been coincidental that the delicately pink 'blush-rose' was the flower which typically appeared. If it were not natural flowers it would be artificial. They appeared in sugar paste on the sides of the cake, and in a vase on top, often with foliage trailing down around the body of the cake and emphasising the elevated overall effect.

By the 1880s, however, 'virgin purity' (Marchant 1879: 81) was exercising a powerful fascination and a cult of whiteness had set in. Not only were wedding cakes to be white-iced – that was agreed by all – but any trace of colour was to be eliminated from flower decorations and even from foliage. Confectioners might find it monotonous – a strong protest appeared in *The British Baker* in 1887 – but there was nothing they could do: by then only white flowers were to be used and the world was to be scoured for suitably white varieties. The green of their foliage and of added ferns was at first allowable but even these were progressively eliminated. Uniformity of the whites used became an important criterion in judging decorative schemes, and this was the period at which piping, known for a generation, was taken up with enthusiasm. It allowed the creation of an entirely formal style of decoration in exactly the same icing as the main covering of the cake, of exactly the same white therefore. The demand for exact matching on a purely piped cake tended then to exclude any other kind of ornamentation. It even held back for perhaps a decade the adoption of pillars to raise the cake since these were bound to infringe the uniform purity of the white piped form. As a key symbolic element in the ensemble of the white wedding, with the bride's dress and veil, the cake became definitionally and meaningfully white for a generation at least. There was no question of the confectioners of Edinburgh, with their pink cakes, standing against an idea whose time had so conclusively come.

A final more tentative point to note about the classic cake relates it to gender. The pretty mid-Victorian cake with blush-roses around it, as pictured in an early edition by Mrs Beeton (1872), can perhaps be seen as intentionally relating to the bride in her femininity, a bride who was to identify with the cake by herself cutting it at the wedding breakfast. The piped style which replaced it did not strike the same chord: it was created and propagated by men, it petrified fluid forms, denatured natural ones and drained away colour, to make something splendid and amazing in its skill but, as far as its form was concerned, without immediate emotional relevance. There was nothing which could apparently be construed as feminine, nor, it is tempting to say, human at all. An iceberg was a not inappropriate metaphor for its cold impersonality.[5]

MARRIAGE IN THE NINETEENTH CENTURY AND THE CLASSIC CAKE

The classic cake as it developed was therefore explicitly and meaningfully white. Each specimen corresponded uniquely to a particular wedding – it was *the* wedding cake – but it avoided what might have been expected, the obvious forms of individuation adopted for other cakes made at the same period for particular people and events. Its decoration was notably impersonal, standardised and perhaps masculine, at least not feminine. What had this to do with marriage as it developed in the nineteenth century? Was there a relationship here between the marriages being made at weddings and this strange quasi-food object developing for them?

In the first place the classic cake makes the point for us who can now read it through the contrast with our own present that, whatever the personal relationship of the couple marrying, the marriage that they were entering was externally defined. This was particularly true for the middle classes for whom respectability was a leading and much identified preoccupation. Perkin (1989: 90; cf. Dyhouse 1978: 87–8) portrays this section of the society as the bearers of an evangelical Christian ideology and emerging in the nineteenth century as the moral leaders for the nation. It was for them and by them, rather than for either the upper or the working classes, that the wedding styles and cakes which would be carried forward and generalised to the entire population in the twentieth century were formed. For couples of this class, though their weddings were experienced as unique for themselves, what they were subscribing to in getting married was a heavily sanctioned common pattern. This the essentially uniform cake accurately symbolised.

What the cake and its context in the white wedding[6] marked, however, was more than just this commonality. The distinctive pattern now appears to have been particularly to do with the increasing unease with the sexuality of marriage. In a long-term shift from a pre-Reformation world in which the final stage of official religious procedures of marriage was often the visit of the priest to bless the bridal chamber, and indeed the bed with the couple in it, and in contrast to attitudes even in the nineteenth century amongst both the aristocracy and the 'rough' working class, for the respectable it became increasingly difficult to embrace the sexual implications of marriage with an open and straightforward enthusiasm. Perkin describes how an 'ideal of female passionlessness dominated public discourse on sexuality' from the 1820s onwards. 'Public writing maintained that overt sexuality was demeaning in the "nice" middle-class woman.' Sex was 'civilised', she asserts, by excluding it from the attention of the young to the greatest extent possible; 'virginity being the most prized virtue in a middle-class bride', mothers did their best to keep their daughters in a state of apprehensive ignorance (Perkin 1989: 276–7). Such ignorance was not exclusively female either (Harrison 1977: 3ff.). It may contain an element of exaggeration to write, as Perkin does, that 'ignorance of sex started off many middle-class marriages in an atmosphere of horror for each partner' (Perkin 1989: 3), but the generation of a problem over the making of marriages is clear. There was at best a tricky and often embarrassing transition to be made from the single life in which virginity had become such a supreme value, to a married state in which it would have to be, ever so privately, given up. As Dyhouse reports: 'the essence of femininity was defined as purity, and little girls should appear innocent, virginal, and unsullied in every way. Dressed in white muslin frills, they were abjured to keep clean, to keep quiet, and to keep still' (1981: 23). The little girls had somehow to become married women.

The problem was not new; in the eighteenth century it was one of the factors which had led to a progressive withdrawing of respectable marriage-making from the public gaze (Stone 1992: 25–9), but for the ever larger, respectable middle classes in the nineteenth century, weddings could no longer hide. This, combined with a heightening preoccupation with virginity and sexual purity, produced the ever-whitening wedding. It was given powerful if unorthodox expression in the 1870s work of the great poet of Victorian married love, Coventry Patmore (1823–96), but in his earlier and most popular work, *The Angel in the House*, which sold more than a quarter of a million copies (de la Mare 1930: xv, 12–13) and came to epitomise the ideal of the Victorian wife, he had already provided a telling literary interpretation of the experience of a wedding. After describing his, or his protagonist's, numbness through the marriage service, he sums up the wedding in four lines:

O, bold seal of a bashful bond,
Which makes the marriage-day to be,
To those before it and beyond,
An iceberg in an Indian sea.
(Patmore 1949)

Writing well before the full elaboration of the white wedding and the cult of virginity, marriage is already experienced as 'a bashful bond', needing to be too boldly sealed. This was a world in which an etiquette book could envisage a woman not being able to face appearing at her own wedding breakfast (Anon. 1854: 32–3). Patmore clearly identifies the source of the uneasiness, and the insight he offers is the more valuable for its rarity. Significantly, in contrast to the present day when every 'soap' has its weddings, when they are a common theme of films, and when videos of the occasion are the latest addition to the money-spinning sequence of ordinary weddings, the Victorian wedding was rarely taken up in novels of the period (cf. Calder 1976: 99, 113 on Dickens). Davidoff and Hall note that 'the open recognition of sexuality . . . was suppressed along with other vulgarities. Male sexual passion was to be contained and hidden, women's to be ignored if not denied. As a result, most records are silent on such subjects' (Davidoff and Hall 1987: 402). And the wedding itself is commonly sucked into the same silence.

It was probably only in the 1880s that the discomfort reached its peak. This was the decade in which both sex and marriage became publicly unavoidable issues for the respectable. It was the decade in which the editor W.T. Stead revealed scandalously in *The Pall Mall Gazette* the details of child prostitution in London, and was convicted in a blaze of publicity for purchasing a 13-year-old as part of a press investigation. Dyhouse finds that this exposé, and the press excitement over the Jack the Ripper murders of young women in London at the end of the decade 'massively increased women's sense of sexual and social vulnerability' and 'fuelled "social purity" movements amongst feminists and others, generating support for vigilance associations, the raising of the age of consent, the policing of prostitution, and "rescue" work of all kinds' (Dyhouse 1989: 166–7). At the same time, marriage itself was an issue: the *Daily Telegraph* ran a summer controversy on the topic 'Is marriage a failure?' and received over 27,000 letters, suggesting clearly the extent of middle-class concern (Rubinstein 1986: 39).

As experienced by a passionate man, the wedding itself had already a generation before been a numbing interlude, cold if brilliant, raised fleetingly between the warmth of happy courtship and – as Patmore was renowned or, in the eyes of some, notorious for seeing it – the glories of the couple's married love in the days ahead. By the time purity and whiteness reached their apogee matters had become a great deal more generally uncomfortable for the respectable, with male lust as well as female virginity and its loss repeatedly brought to the forefront of attention. What is striking, therefore, is that the white wedding emerged not from any supposed Victorian security over marriage and weddings but in a period of acute tensions surrounding them.

This was the context in which the cake assumed its hard, white, genderless, or perhaps masculine but certainly impersonal, decorative surface. It is a context. It is not argued here that the classic cake and the white wedding of which it was a part were functional in any psychological sense, helping individuals through a difficult transition from an asexual single state into a necessarily sexualised relationship in marriage. This was perhaps a problem never resolved as long as the tension over sex remained. Patmore's poetry had become increasingly scandalous for most of his proper readers (Reid 1957: 152), and the event of marriage intensely problematic. The white wedding focused on a veiled bride, symbol of purity, increasingly separated by her characteristic disguise from her own and everyone else's everyday life. It also focused on the cake, similarly white, flower-bedecked and even occasionally veiled. Together they can be seen as a strategy emerging in response to a prevailing situation, marking off the single from the married in typical rite-of-passage style (Van Gennep 1909), but pushing the sexual implications of the transition well away from the public event itself.

MARRIAGE AND CAKES IN THE LATE TWENTIETH CENTURY

By the 1980s almost everything was different. Though some still subscribed to the ideal of confining sex within marriage, the cult of secrecy and virginity were long past. More important, the standard nature of marriage had weakened. A long succession of laws motivated by an intention to remove disabilities from married women and in pursuit of an ideal of equality in marriage had stripped away the bulk of the legal framework which had maintained the once momentous significance of the difference between being single and being married (Charsley 1991: 7–13). For a long time this trend had been to some extent balanced by developing welfare legislation and state benefits predicated on marriage, but under the Conservative government of Mrs Thatcher this too ran out. Despite lip service paid to 'family values', and a real demand that families take greater financial responsibility for their members, taxation and benefit reforms flowed chiefly from the individualistic ideology which Mrs Thatcher famously expressed in her declaration that there is no such thing as 'society'. As fathers and mothers and children, people should individually be responsible for one another, but support, moral and practical, for any idea of the family as a little society founded on marriage was not maintained. A shift in personal taxation from the couple to the individual cut away a residual support for the unity which marriage had sought to create and had once achieved, at least in concept, ideal and law, if never, of course, entirely in practice.

Since the 1980s, whether to marry or 'just' live together has been a matter of rapidly decreasing public moment, a matter for ever-freer individual choice (e.g. Wallace 1987: 160–3). Numbers of weddings declined steeply and when they were celebrated they were commonly either not inaugurating the couple's life together, or were not the first for the parties. What the rules for these new marriages were to be, each couple would need to work out for themselves. In this situation the classic standardising symbolism had become strikingly inappropriate; choice and personal relevance become the new themes.

Already by the early 1980s, the Glasgow study of people setting up their weddings found this way of thinking well established, but its implications for the wedding cake had so far been limited. Despite a history of minor variation which has been sufficiently discussed elsewhere (Charsley 1992), the message the current cake would have delivered to anyone able to read it was still one of the basic standardisation which had been appropriate to a previous age. But a profusion of altogether new styles for cakes was on the point of appearing. Most striking was the arrival of sugar paste, developed primarily in Australia and taken up with enthusiasm in the British sugarcraft movement. This new material being plastic, drapable and delicately mouldable, in contrast to the liquid but hard-setting royal icing previously used, allowed an entirely different style of decoration. It was virtually free of constraints on the shapes which could be covered or formed, and on colours. Naturalistic representation was entirely possible and to that extent encouraged. Applied to the decoration of wedding cakes, it appeared at first chiefly in the form of tablecloth-like coverings, representing the cake as a table on which anything pretty or meaningful, serious or humorous might be set. The long-standing use of artificial flowers on cakes has been noted: these continued to be a major possibility. Previously wax or silk or paper flowers had generally been reduced from their natural complexity to simpler objects which would conform to an overall scheme of decoration, whether white or in colours appropriate to the schemes for the dressing of weddings once the preoccupation with white had faded. Now, in contrast, the new sugarcraft movement developed the skills to allow entirely naturalistic flowers to be produced and it delighted in their elaboration. Instead of either including fresh flowers in the decorative scheme, paying nature a direct compliment, or taking inspiration from the natural in creating decorative artificial forms, a striking subordination of nature is now displayed by its recreation in edible form.[7]

Personalised marriage had finally produced its symbolic counterpart. The classic form of the wedding cake, evolved for Victorian and Edwardian marriages and a standard requirement for them all, has not disappeared but it has been revalued. It has become one option amongst many in an age in which couples are left to work out the rules for themselves. New forms, though they still often use an echo of the old three-tier formula to announce themselves as wedding cakes, otherwise tend to be assimilated to a new category, 'celebration cakes'. Like them they are to be ceremoniously cut and consumed by those assembled to celebrate. A cake in the form of a couple sitting on a settee with the children of their previous partnerships around them, in the form of an old boot with romantic associations, or of the Scottish island on which its laird was marrying his bride (Charsley 1993) became possible for new marriages in the 1990s. The wedding as a personal celebration was flourishing ever more extravagantly, but the change signalled clearly and correctly that, as a distinctive rite of passage making a culturally standardised transition, its end was close.

NOTES

1 ESRC support for Project No. G/00/23/0049 is gratefully acknowledged.
2 Discussion of the evolution of the rich fruit cake and of icing, of cake-breaking and cake-cutting and of much that is not referred to in this paper, as well as documentation for much that is, can be found there. Referencing for historical sources is, in the light of its availability there, not generally reproduced here.
3 This evidence concerns the republishing of her recipe by another author and her apparent challenge to it (Charsley 1992: 56).
4 The impetus for returning to the topic of the wedding cake was initially provided by a conference of the Design History Society held in Glasgow in December 1994, entitled 'Design for Selling', at which the first version of this chapter was presented.
5 But see also Charsley (1987: 105–8).
6 The familiar expression seems not to have become established until well into the twentieth century.
7 The fascination in Europe with edible reproductions of often inedible objects goes back at least to the subtleties of the late medieval period. It has taken a variety of forms: see James (1982), Charsley (1992: 37–41, 64–5). However, as James later commented, confectionery remains 'a relatively undigested area of food study' (James 1990: 671).

REFERENCES

Anon. (1854) *Etiquette, Social Ethics and the Courtesies of Society*, London: Orr.
Beeton, I. (1872) *Beeton's Every-day Cookery and Housekeeping Book*, London: Ward Lock.
British Baker (1887) 'How to colour cakes', *British Baker*, February: 16.
Caird, J. (1809) *The Complete Confectioner and Family Cook*, Leith.
Calder, J. (1976) *Women and Marriage in Victorian Fiction*, London: Thames and Hudson.
Charsley, S.R. (1987) 'Interpretation and custom: the case of the wedding cake', *Man* (N.S.) 22: 93–110.
—— (1991) *Rites of Marrying, The Wedding Industry in Scotland*, Manchester: Manchester University Press.
—— (1992) *Wedding Cakes and Cultural History*, London: Routledge.
—— (1993) 'The rise of the British wedding cake', *Natural History* 102, 12: 58–67.
Davidoff, L. and Hall, C. (1987) *Family Fortunes. Men and Women of the English Middle Class, 1780–1850*, London: Hutchinson.
de la Mare, W. (ed.) (1930) *The Eighteen-Eighties. Essays*, Cambridge: Cambridge University Press.
Dods, M. (1833) *Cook and Housewife's Manual*, new edn, Edinburgh: Oliver and Boyd.
Dyhouse, C. (1978) 'The condition of England 1860–1900', in L. Lerner (ed.) *The Victorians*, New York: Holmes and Meier.

—— (1981) *Girls Growing Up in Late Victorian and Edwardian England*, London: Routledge.

—— (1989) *Feminism and the Family in England 1880–1939*, Oxford: Blackwell.

Frazer, Mrs (1806) *Practice of Cookery, Pastry and Confectionery*, 5th edn, Edinburgh: Hill.

Gommez, R. (1899) *Cake Decoration: Flower and Classic Piping*, London: *Baker and Confectioner*.

Harrison, F. (1977) *The Dark Angel. Aspects of Victorian Sexuality*, London: Sheldon Press.

Henisch, B.A. (1984) *Cakes and Characters: An English Christmas Tradition*, London: Prospect Books.

James, A. (1982) 'Confections, concoctions and conceptions', in B. Waites, T. Bennett and G. Martin (eds) *Popular Culture: Past and Present*, London: Croom Helm.

—— (1990) 'The good, the bad and the delicious: the role of confectionery in British society', *Sociological Review* 38: 666–88.

Marchant, W.T. (1879) *Betrothals and Bridals, with a Chat about Wedding Cakes and Wedding Customs*, London: Hill.

Oxford English Dictionary, Compact Edition (1971) Oxford: Oxford University Press.

Patmore, C. (1949) *The Poems of Coventry Patmore* (edited and with an Introduction, F. Page), London: Oxford University Press.

Perkin, J. (1989) *Women and Marriage in Nineteenth-Century England*, London: Routledge.

Raffald, E. (1769) *The Experienced English Housekeeper*, Manchester: the Author.

Reid, J.C. (1957) *The Mind and Art of Coventry Patmore*, London: Routledge.

Rubinstein, D. (1986) *Before the Suffragettes. Women's Emancipation in the 1890s*, Brighton: Harvester.

Stone, L. (1992) *Uncertain Unions. Marriage in England 1660–1753*, Oxford: Oxford University Press.

Van Gennep, A. (1909) *Les Rites de passage*, Paris: Nourry.

Wallace, C. (1987) *For Richer, For Poorer. Growing Up in and Out of Work*, London: Tavistock.

Youngson, A.J. (1966) *The Making of Classical Edinburgh 1750–1840*, Edinburgh: Edinburgh University Press.

Chapter 4

How British is British food?

Allison James

Since Elizabeth David first published her book about Mediter-ranean cooking in 1950, four years before food rationing ended, the reticence and conservatism of the British palate appears to have been in sharp decline (Mennell 1985).[1] The cookery columns which had become regular features in newspapers and magazines by the 1950s gave way to a more serious form of food journalism in the 1960s and, since the mid-1970s, specialist radio and television, which have food as their topic, have begun to be broadcast. Amidst this burgeoning industry, interest in 'foreign' food seemed by the 1990s to have emerged triumphant: chicken tikka was recorded as a favoured filling for the British Rail sandwich, and chicken tikka masala, chilli con carne and lasagne had become bestsellers in Tesco's pre-cooked food range (*The Sunday Times* 23 September 1991).

But although these trends might seem to indicate that an irrevocable change in British food traditions had taken place, by the early 1990s there were also signs of movement in the opposite direction. Alongside the enthusiasm for 'foreign' food was an increased parochialising of taste, as evidenced in the loud champi-oning of 'gutsy, unpretentious' food (Bati 1991) and the flotation of Harry Ramsden's fish and chip shop on the Stock Exchange (Young 1989).

This chapter explores these apparent changes in the patterning of food preferences in Britain through examining representations of food to be found in the popular press in the early 1990s – newspapers, magazines and food journalism – and considers what kind of impact foreign food could be said to be having on British food traditions at that time. Did it register a massive dislocation in food habits, so that now it is no longer possible for the British to identify culturally with the food they eat, or was there, instead, a more subtle continuity occurring which was working to reaffirm a sense of what is truly British food?

FOOD AND IDENTITY

A long and respectable tradition of anthropological work on social and animal classification has established that food marks out cultural identities. Simple equations such as 'we eat meat, they don't', 'we eat horse, they don't', 'they eat insects, we don't', affirm, in shared patterns of consumption and shared notions of edibility, our difference from others (see, for example, Bulmer 1967, Lévi-Strauss 1962). Indeed, these prejudices and persuasions may map on to and be given further cogency by the patterning of our behaviour in other domains, from household management through to sexual liaisons and social intimacies (Tambiah 1969, Leach 1964, Douglas 1975). It is surely the roast beef of old England that unconsciously sustains the feeling of incipient British nationalism which floods to the surface when unarticulated cultural stereotypes of the Japanese are wittily reaffirmed in British newspaper assertions that they eat anything. Under the headline, 'Ravenous Japanese stone the crows' we learn that in the coastal town of Kisakata one solution to pest control for Japanese farmers has been the incorporation of crow meat into their diet (*Guardian*, 16 November 1991). More poignantly, it is the same roast beef of old England which the continuing crisis over BSE threatens; not merely an outrage to the British meat industry, it menaces a core symbol of national identity. And so it is that in parlour games and pub quizzes we are asked to affirm that lasagne comes from Italy, chow mein from China and goulash from Hungary: a seemingly fixed culinary order sustains and stakes out fixed cultural identities.

Such stereotyping, as ever, contradicts the evidence of a tremendous diversity of food preferences within any particular culture, a diversity which sustains not only regional specialities but also often a more localised than nationalised food tradition. Nonetheless, in the popular imagination, and in popular food writing, there is such a thing as 'Spanish cooking' or 'German food' and it is precisely through the continual promulgation of such food stereotypes that we get to 'know' what 'Italian' or 'Indian' food *should* consist of in our encounters with foreign food. Indeed, food is one of the primary ways in which notions of 'otherness' are articulated.[2] As

Zubaida (1992) notes for the Middle East, gastro-nationalism is an important resource for identity marking:

> Communities were always proud of their own food while denigrating that of their opponents or rivals, often in terms of stereotypes.... Mosulis are ridiculed by Baghdadis for allegedly putting garlic in everything. Another common traditional theme is that of generosity vs. meanness. I have heard, in the old days, Baghdadi women and cooks jeer at Syrians ... for being very economical with meat: all those salads and pastes that were just being introduced in Iraq, *tabbouleh*, *hommous*, *baba-ghanoush*, were only means of saving meat. In contrast 'we' cooked lots of meat in grills and stews.
>
> (Zubaida 1992: 19)

Yet despite this apparent certainty of what 'we' and 'they' eat, there is also a fickleness in the way in which food, in practice, sustains images of cultural identity. First, some awkward historical facts challenge the very idea of there being a traditional relationship between food, culture and identity. Cuisines are not limited by geography or nationhood. Each national cuisine bears the traces of trade, travel and, increasingly, of technology, so that food could more correctly be said to be constitutive of global rather than local cultures (Mennell 1985, Mintz 1985). It was, for instance, only at the end of the nineteenth century that 'traditional Provençal cooking' became dominated by olive oil (Goody 1982). Prior to that it was but sparingly used. Similarly, Zubaida notes that the recent emergence of the 'standard Mediterranean diet' – olive oil, garlic and sun-dried tomatoes – masks the variation within the region and is:

> a modern construction of food writers and publicists in western Europe and North America earnestly preaching what is now thought to be a healthy diet to their audiences by invoking a stereotype of the healthy other on the shores of the Mediterranean. Their colleagues in Mediterranean countries are only too willing to perpetuate this myth. The fact of the matter is that the Mediterranean contains varied cultures and that Spain is in a minority of regions (the others are Greece and southern Italy) which use olive oil as a predominant medium of cooking.
>
> (Zubaida 1992: 23)

A second challenge to the presumed role of food as a cultural marker of national identity arises from the ways in which, *within* any local culture, it is also used extensively to register ideas of difference and, in particular, gradations of status. Again, this has been well documented in the traditional anthropological literature (see Fieldhouse 1986 for an extensive account) and histories of diet (Drummond and Wilbraham 1991 [1939], Tannahill 1973). For instance, in most cultures, rites of passage which mark changes of social status and hence identity are accompanied by special kinds of food or rules about its consumption. Within British culture, for example, marriage is traditionally marked by a special feast whose finale is the white, tiered wedding cake (Charsley 1987, this volume) while among the LoDagaa of northern Ghana, on the other hand, everyday foodstuffs become invested with particular rules restricting their consumption during rites of passage such as funeral ceremonies (Goody 1982). Note has also been taken in the literature of the way in which gender and age are signified through food, with women and young children in particular being prescribed or proscribed special foodstuffs (Fieldhouse 1986).

Paradoxically, then, food provides a fluid symbolic medium for making statements about identity. Through the invocation of sets of inflexible cultural stereotypes, particular foodstuffs are linked to particular localised as well as nationalised or, indeed, globalised identities (James 1996). What I eat may reveal that I am English or Cornish, a Hindu or a Jew, a child or an adult or an international traveller or trendsetter. It may, also, more prosaically, indicate my social class and status, as Bourdieu (1989) has shown in his discussion of class distinctions in France. He suggests that the choices people make over what they eat reproduce symbolically their class position. Though income may appear to be a determining factor in what people eat Bourdieu dismisses the notion that such purely economic explanations account for class differences and convincingly demonstrates, through detailed statistical and epidemiological analysis, that it is ideas of cultural taste about what constitutes proper food which work to perpetuate class divisions and lifestyles. Rising incomes do not, he argues, necessarily alter people's consumption patterns noting, for example, that clerical workers spend less on food than manual workers both in absolute and relative terms. Explanations for class differences between what people eat must be sought, therefore, through the wider appreciation of ideas of cultural taste:

In the face of the new ethic for sobriety for the sake of slimness, which is most recognised at the highest levels of the social hierarchy, peasants and especially industrial workers maintain an ethic of convivial indulgence. A bon vivant is not just someone who enjoys eating and drinking; he is someone capable of entering into the generous and familiar . . . relationship that is encouraged and symbolised by eating and drinking together, in a conviviality which sweeps away restraints and reticence.

(Bourdieu 1989: 179)

Thus it is that the senior executive at a restaurant chooses a light grill, while the industrial worker favours more substantial dishes and finishes the meal with both cheese *and* dessert.

In this chapter it is this 'otherness' of class and status with which I shall be mostly concerned through a consideration of the kinds of impact which foreign food is having on the traditional markers of class and status in the British diet. Though, as Goody (1982) notes, this is not a necessary feature of all cuisines, this chapter will argue that in Britain food has always served as a marker of class and continues to do so.

FOOD, STATUS AND CLASS

Mennell (1985) notes that within the British food tradition the relationship between food and social class identity is complexly marked and observes that, by the nineteenth century, British class identity had ironically begun to be mediated through (foreign) French food. In contrast to the highly elaborate cuisine which had developed in French court society during the seventeenth and eighteenth centuries, the British gentry had continued to live off their land, eating simple dressed meats and puddings. During the nineteenth century, however, there developed an increased culinary dependency on France as the elite abandoned traditional British fare and country cooking and adopted French cooks and French cuisine:

while the continuity in development in French *haute cuisine* from the eighteenth century into the nineteenth is quite clear, a coarsening and decline of the great English 'farmhouse' tradition of the eighteenth century is rather apparent in the nineteenth. Quite apart from any effects which rapid industrialisation may have had in disrupting that tradition, its vitality was probably sapped by the dominance which French models enjoyed at the highest level of society. English cookery was, so to speak, decapitated.

(Mennell 1985: 135)

It was a gastronomic hegemony by the French which extended over most of Europe, and North America as well, and, writing in the 1930s, Drummond and Wilbraham note its influence in the ways in which courses for a meal became structured:

The French fashion in the arrangement of the courses at dinner, adopted by the wealthy classes in the eighteenth century, remained popular throughout the following century.

One connoisseur held that:

It is a bad dinner when there are not at least five varieties: a substantial dish of fish, one of meat, one of game, one of poultry and, above all, a ragout with truffles. . . . They form the absolute minimum and *sine qua non* of a dinner for one person.

(1991 [1939]: 337)

However, although by the late 1800s the food of the elite and aspiring upper middle-class British families therefore had a distinctly French flavour, there was at least one line of resistance to the influence of foreign food. As Mennell notes, the cooking of average middle-class people 'remained largely untouched by such influences' (1985: 206). Indeed, Mennell argues, this foreign influence seems to have been fiercely resisted well into the twentieth century and was an attitude which 'formed a dyke, somewhere in the middle ranks of the social hierarchy, through which fashionable French models did not seep' (1985: 206). Furthermore, for the poor, food was both monotonous and low in nutrition, a far cry from the abundant table of the rich. Drummond and Wilbraham describe the diet of factory workers in Lancashire in the 1860s as follows:

records of the diets of the Lancashire operatives in 1864 show that they lived largely on bread, oatmeal, bacon, a very little butter, treacle, tea and coffee. Cheap jams made their appearance on the market in the 'eighties and immediately became very popular. Most of them contained very little of the fruit they were alleged to be made from and were simply concoctions made from the cheapest fruit or vegetable pulp obtainable, coloured and flavoured as required. Their sweetness made them very popular with poor families: bread and jam became the chief food of poor children for two meals out of three.

(1991 [1939]: 332)

This is not to say that for the lower classes in France a similar disparity was not in evidence. The important difference, however, is that in Britain class status and high distinction were dependent on the adoption of a *French*, rather than a British, gastronomic style. It did not merely reflect greater access by the rich to more abundant and varied foodstuffs.[3]

Thus, historically, within the British food tradition foreign food has worked to bring about both change and continuity in food preferences through different mobilisations of class identity. The following analysis of contemporary representations of foreign food will show that this 'making a difference' is, in itself, a kind of continuity in British food traditions. Thus, although broadly concurring with Mennell's assertion that the twentieth century has seen a progressive uniformity in food consumption across the social classes in Britain, I shall show that, nonetheless, subtle markers of difference in relation to eating foreign food still persist as reminders of class difference, as revealed in contemporary popular publications about food.

FOREIGN FOOD VS. BRITISH FOOD

In many of the 'foodie' magazines,[4] which are now widely available in newsagents and on supermarket shelves, there is a constant promotion of a particular kind of foreign fare which, I suggest, has a particular audience in view. The pages of *Good Housekeeping* and *Good Food* magazines, for example, are filled with recipes and detailed descriptions of food and wine which image the foreignness of foreign countries and lifestyles. In the early 1990s regular readers of *Good Food* could, in the travellers' tastes section, sample Greece (April 1993), India (May 1993) and Tunisia (June 1993) on a monthly basis. Reflecting popular television series, such as those hosted by Keith Floyd on France and Spain, these articles were aimed largely at an upper middle-class readership, with the time, money and aspirations to indulge in such fantasies. Such popular magazines offered what amounted to a form of literary and culinary expatriate cosmopolitanism, which stressed the necessity for authenticity in the replication of foreign cuisines through an exact and exacting detailing of recipes.[5]

Similar claims could be found in other contemporaneous food writing and in the food journalism by now common in the quality press (see also Levy 1986, Davidson 1988). These foodie writers sought and found authenticity in the small scale, the subtly spiced, the delicately flavoured foods of foreign fields. Reported in the food columns of weekend broadsheet newspapers and described and enacted on television by food experts, it was a form of cultural authenticity through food which was being bought and cooked. For example, in their book, *A Mediterranean Harvest*, published in 1987, Scaravelli and Cohen suggest that their readers buy a range of cooking oils in order to be able to reproduce the authentic regional tastes of the Mediterranean: extra virgin olive oil, virgin olive oil, olive oil, corn oil, sunflower oil and peanut oil. Although to have such a wide variety may seem unnecessarily extravagant, Scaravelli and Cohen argue that 'each oil is distinctive and each has a particular use' (1987: 18). In this way the reader is encouraged to reproduce these foreign dishes at home as authentically as possible. This is classy food for those with class aspirations and it reflected the ever-increasing ease with which foreign ingredients were becoming available to the British consumer. For example, Delia Smith's recipes – the nation's favourite cookery writer, her summer collection book being reprinted eight times when it was first published in 1993 – are liberally sprinkled with ingredients and recipes foreign to traditional English cookery: red peppers (Italy), halloumi cheese (Greece), fontina cheese (Italy), tabouleh salad (Middle East), fattoush salad (Middle East), buffalo mozzarella cheese (Italy), lemon grass (Thailand), Californian grilled fish (America), chorizo sausage (Spain) and Sri Lankan curry (Sri Lanka).

Selling over 5 million copies of her cookery books, Delia Smith is described as the 'Mrs Beeton of our times'.[6] And it was, of course, Isabella Beeton whose *Book of Household Management* (1861), was, as Mennell notes, responsible for giving urban lower middle-class and middle-class women in Britain the confidence and knowledge to cook good British food. But although in Mrs Beeton's food 'there are superficial signs of French influence', it is mainly 'plain English', with the recipes demonstrating an unequivocal lack of development in cooking styles (1985: 214). Mennell's somewhat gloomy conclusion is that:

with the exception of [Eliza Acton], it does not seem unfair to describe the food of the nineteenth-century English domestic cookery books as rather monotonous, and above all lacking any sense of the *enjoyment* of food.

(1985: 214)

To call Delia Smith the new Mrs Beeton would seem, then, a curious parallel to draw, unless, that is, by the early 1990s there was no longer such a thing as British food?

BRITISH FOOD VS. FOREIGN FOOD

In direct and apparent contrast to this patterning of food preferences, which would seem to suggest a waning of British food, another trend can be seen emerging within contemporary British food writing of the early 1990s that points in the opposite direction. It might well be called 'food nostalgia'. Within this movement, the many local and regional gastronomic traditions to be found within the British Isles are celebrated and brought to the nation's wider attention. A newspaper report in 1991 – somewhat tongue in cheek – remarked this development, in its reporting of a court case involving a a Stilton cheese. In the face of the threat to standardise and regulate cheese production images of tradition, continuity and the nation's heritage are rallied in defence:

A mature Stilton cheese, whose mites and maggots were such that Daniel Defoe said a spoon was needed to eat them has won a legal battle over hygiene. . . . The small residents were essential to genuine Stilton said Adrian Williams, solicitor for Safeways supermarket, rather than evidence of careless cheese-handling. He accused the trading standards officers of ignorance. 'Here is a product which has been English to the bone from the 1700s onwards', he said. 'It has had mites on it ever since.' The bench dismissed the case. Peter Pugson, chairman of the UK Cheese Guild called the decision 'a victory for English common sense' and offered the standards department a place on the guild's diploma course.

(Wainwright 1991)

In a similar vein, each year the food experts from the *Guardian* newspaper set off in search of the great British banger, sampling hundreds of locally produced sausages, manufactured for the large part by small family butchers in rural communities. In the BBC *Good Food* magazine were listed the names and addresses of specialist food shops and local retail outlets where traditional, regional British food might be purchased.

Such activity is a far cry from salsas and sauces. It would seem to bear witness to the revival of traditional British fare, to mark the resurrection of the country cooking abandoned by the gentry in the eighteenth and nineteenth centuries when they turned to a more French style of cuisine. In what can be seen as an anxious response to the seeming culinary fragmentation of contemporary British society, food writers within this tradition were lamenting the increasing foreignness of British food:

> The British, it seems, have got the food they deserve. Having shamefully neglected our own traditional dishes for 40 years, we now have a flashy, meretricious cuisine based, for the most part, on ersatz imitations of Mediterranean foods, unrelated to any even in our own history.
>
> (Boxer 1991: 32)

For Boxer, truly British food comprises roast meats and vegetables, stews, pies and pasties, rounded off with the stodgy bland food epitomised by steamed puddings. These dishes, as described by Bati, were in the 1990s making a fashion comeback:

> For the past 10 years too many chefs have been mucking about with food. Now they're learning how to get flavour out of cheap ingredients. And the public is ready for food their mothers have forgotten how to cook – gutsy, unpretentious food.
>
> (Antony Worrall-Thompson, quoted in Bati 1991)

However, as with the desire to reproduce authentic foreign food at home or to eat out in restaurants specialising in particular regional cuisines, any individual's access to this celebration of quality, diversity, tradition and authenticity was limited. Bati's (1991) location of this food discourse was primarily in London: in Simpson's-in-the-Strand, Porters in Covent Garden, Green's in St James, Boyd's in Kensington and just a few provincial restaurants named as exemplars. Like the foodies' celebration of the distinctiveness of regional foreign cuisines, this is not, on the whole, the provenance of mass consumerism, family food purchasing or of large-scale supermarket shopping. Neither is it suited to quick snacks and Sunday dinners. Time is required to seek out, purchase and prepare the necessary specialised ingredients, and to patronise restaurants starred for particular cuisines can be expensive. Here, too, then, the targeted market niche was that of the upper middle class. It is, therefore, with some irony I note that Staffordshire oatcakes (a breakfast item purchased by an earlier generation of my own family of male workers in the mining and pottery industries and female workers in service for the wealthy) could in 1992 be bought mail order – but at a price (*Good Food*, November 1992).[7]

FOOD CREOLISATION

It would seem therefore that the embrace of both foreign food and the emergence of a food nostalgia did not represent an emergent gastronomic pluralism in Britain in the early 1990s. Neither did it register a change in food consumption practices in relation to class. Food, whether foreign or British, continued to speak to older class divides and thus the apparent diversity which these two trends incorporated masked a hidden unity: such foods were only to be enjoyed by the few rather than the many, which means that the twin embrace of foreign food and traditional foods were simply recreating, reordering or sustaining old social divisions along class and educational lines. It is, after all, the *fact* of difference which really makes a difference.

But what, then, can be made of the apparently contradictory evidence, noted at the outset, that foreign food would now appear to be food for the masses, widely available, readily consumed and that by 1992 Indian take-aways outnumbered that most traditional of traditional British institutions, the fish and chip shop (Mintel International 1992)? Alternatively, what might be made of the observation that pasta is now seen as British, rather than Italian, fare?[8] One answer lies in considering what exactly, in terms of the British mass market, now counts as foreign food. Turning once more to an examination of media representations of food in the early 1990s, some clues can be found but this time attention is given to the food journalism aimed at a more mass market.

In a series of articles on Provence and Provençal cooking in the *Radio Times* (produced to accompany the television serialisation of Peter Mayle's book, *A Year in Provence*) the mass public of distrusting, fearful ordinary British people have to be tempted into trying out foreign food with sets of careful and personalised step-by-step instructions (*Radio Times* 6–12 and 13–19 March

1993). French meals have to be quick and easy to prepare if they are to be eaten in Britain. But, after the first two weeks, the pudding recipes signalled the end of this gastronomic adventure and bore witness to the return of a more familiar puritanical, traditional British style. Although 'Mireille Johnston, author of the BBC's French Cookery Course, rounded off her selection of Provençal recipes with two delicious desserts', only one seems to be a 'refreshingly fruity' French dessert. The other has more than a hint of a British pudding about it: it is described as 'sinfully sweet', recalling the 'naughty but nice' attitude to sweetness which, as I have described elsewhere (James 1990), is a decidedly British characteristic. In France no food is sinful.

This subtle distinction, heralding a British-like Provençal cooking, exemplifies then a third contemporary food trend in Britain: food creolisation. Now ironically seen as a new tradition, the Cafe Lazeez on the Old Brompton Road epitomised this movement in the early 1990s, describing its dishes – the Frontier burger, for example – as 'a sophisticated and mouth-watering melange of the East with the West, illustrating the culinary style that has evolved in the UK over the past 30 years' (quoted in Brown 1993). Brown described the cafe as 'the least Indian of all the Indian restaurants I have ever visited', with its Australian *maître d'*, English waitresses, Italian-style decor, gold Indian-style spherical artefacts and Pakistani cuisine (Brown 1993). The food was likewise a cultural blending: 'they cut down on ghee and chilli in Indian dishes, and . . . they Indianise thoroughly western dishes such as burgers, tuna and lamb chops' (Brown 1993).

This food trend is also remarked on by Timothy Mo in his novel, *Sour Sweet*, which relates the settling in of a Chinese family into the British way of life as proprietors of a take-away food establishment:

> The food they sold, certainly wholesome, nutritious, colourful, even tasty in its way, had been researched by Chen. It bore no resemblance at all to Chinese cuisine. They served from a stereotyped menu, similar to those outside countless other establishments in the UK. . . . 'Sweet and sour pork' was their staple, naturally: batter musket balls encasing a tiny core of meat, laced with a scarlet sauce that had an interesting effect on the urine of the consumer the next day. Chen knew because he tried some and almost fainted with shock the morning after,

fearing some frightful internal haemorrhaging. . . . 'Spare ribs' (what ever they were) also seemed popular. So were spring rolls, basically a Northerner's snack, which Lily parsimoniously filled mostly with beansprouts.

(Mo 1992: 105–6)

For Lily, Chen's wife, such food preferences serve to confirm her suspicions about the English: 'English taste buds must be as degraded as their care of their parents' (1992: 105).

Partly, of course, this amalgam of tastes and cuisines represents an accommodation to local conditions and ingredients as the popular Indian food writer Madhur Jaffrey (1982) has suggested. She began her cooking career in student digs in London, where she endeavoured to recapture the taste of India. Recipes sent from home had to be adapted to local conditions so that, in her Indian cookery book a stand-by recipe is called 'pork chipolatas cooked in an Indian style' (1982: 61). However, the willing and enthusiastic acceptance in Britain of such creolised food traditions – seen in the canned and instant products on supermarket shelves and the menus of fast food take-aways – may, in the light of the earlier discussion, indicate rather more than a simple pragmatism. Ironically, it may be a new mark of Britishness through its accommodation under a foreign guise of traditional British attitudes to food and cooking. Mennell notes, for example, that a common feature of British attitudes to food is a concern with saving both time and money (1985: 260–1). As noted previously, food in Britain, being regarded traditionally more as a necessity than a pleasure, means that the emphasis in food writing and recipes is often laid on no-nonsense, economical cooking. British food is food you can trust, quick and easy to prepare, wholesome and nutritious. As Mennell (1985) observes, convenience and frozen foods were readily embraced by the British in the 1960s. They provided ways to save time, to make 'posher nosh' with cheating 'means' (Mennell 1985: 260).

The enthusiastic acceptance of creolised foreign food aimed at a mass market thus represents, I suggest, a continuity, rather than a diminution, of the Britishness of British food traditions, for in the take-away or pre-prepared products aimed at the mass food market these quintessentially British attitudes are but thinly veiled. A spoonful of pesto, a packet of pasta, or a bottle of cook-in-sauce can be seen as simply one way to spice up plain British mince, rather than as registering a desire to cook authentic Italian food. Eating curry as a new sauce for chips and pot noodles as an alternative to a sandwich does not mean that the British are embracing culinary diversity; it is simply old food habits in a new form.

CONCLUSION

The changes which Mennell (1985) notes as having occurred in British food – the shift towards an increasing uniformity of food preferences across social classes alongside an increased variation in the kinds of food being eaten – are therefore, I would suggest, tempered by some rather more subtle continuities which carry on marking out British food as British. First, as this chapter has argued, distinctions of taste continue to serve as markers of class difference (Bourdieu 1989). No longer conceived simply in terms of a willingness to reject traditional British fare in favour of more classy foreign food, status is now being displayed through recourse to notions of authenticity. Be this in relation to foreign or British food, the time and/or money needed for such display of style is what provides the lines of class distinction. Alternatively, the consumption of traditional British fare may be the new high-status distinction, in contrast to the more readily available take-away, ersatz dishes of southern Europe, China and India which anyone can consume. Authenticity, after all, must have its price.

Second, and somewhat contradictorily, Britishness may be continuing to be marked out in the appearance and ready acceptance of creolised foreign food: bearing the traditional British culinary markers of a concern with saving time and money, creolised food is, ironically, a kind of foreign food which characterises what is truly British about contemporary food consumption in Britain.

NOTES

1 My use of the term 'British' here overrides, of course, traditional regional variations between dietary practices in England, Wales and Scotland as discussed below. However, for the purposes of the argument presented here concerning class and status such differences can, I suggest, be elided.

2 Many popular cookery books follow this tradition. Their titles make claims to presenting Italian food, Greek cookery, etc. and rarely acknowledge the tremendous culinary diversity to be found within those countries.

3 Bourdieu's (1989) point is that in France distinctions between classes are made in terms of the types of food eaten. Though these are different they do not represent a transgression of something which might be called 'French' food.
4 Alan Davidson is described by Paul Levy as 'the leader of the British Scholar Foodies' (1984: 126). He was the inspiration behind the annual British foodie event, the Oxford Symposium on Food at St Anthony's College, which held its first meeting in 1979.
5 As DeVault (1991) has shown, although the lower middle classes might aspire to such cooking they are unlikely to put it into practice.
6 This description can be found on the book jacket.
7 By 1996 oatcakes have become more widely known and are now available in some supermarkets.
8 Personal communication from Pat Caplan. Ongoing research in London reveals that informants under the age of 40 do not regard pasta as a foreign dish but have incorporated it into their culinary repertoire.

REFERENCES

Bati, A. (1991) 'Britannia rules the waves', *Sunday Times*, 22 September.
Beeton, I. (1861) *Beeton's Book of Household Management*, London: S. Beeton.
Bourdieu, P. (1989) *Distinction*, London: Routledge and Kegan Paul.
Boxer, A. (1991) 'Whatever happened to British food?' *Sunday Times*, 22 September.
Brown, C. (1993) 'Prawn again', *Sunday Times*, 9 May.
Bulmer, R. (1967) 'Why is the cassowary not a bird? A problem of zoological taxonomy among the Karam of the New Guinea Highlands', *Man* (N.S.) 2, 1: 5–25.
Charsley, S. (1987) 'Interpretation and custom: the case of the wedding cake', *Man* (N.S.) 22, 2: 93–110.
Davidson, A. (1988) *A Kipper with My Tea*, London: Macmillan.
DeVault, M.L. (1991) *Feeding the Family: The Social Organisation of Caring as Gendered Work*, Chicago, Ill.: University of Chicago Press.
Douglas, M. (1975) 'Deciphering a meal', in M. Douglas (ed.) *Implicit Meanings*, London: Routledge and Kegan Paul.
Drummond, J.C. and Wilbraham, A.S. (1991) [1939] *The Englishman's Food: Five Centuries of English Diet*, London: Pimlico.
Fieldhouse, P. (1986) *Food and Nutrition: Customs and Culture*, London: Croom Helm.
Goody, J. (1982) *Cooking, Cuisine and Class*, Cambridge: Cambridge University Press.
Jaffrey, M. (1982) *Indian Cookery*, London: BBC Publications.
James, A. (1990) 'The good, the bad and the delicious: the role of confectionery in British society', *Sociological Review* 38, 4: 666–88.
—— (1996) 'Cooking the books: global or local identities in contemporary British food cultures', in D. Howes (ed.) *Cross-cultural Consumption: Global Markets and Local Realities*, London: Routledge.

Leach, E. (1964) 'Anthropological aspects of language: animal categories and verbal abuse', in E.H. Lennenberg (ed.) *New Directions in the Study of Language*, Cambridge, Mass.: MIT Press.

Lévi-Strauss, C. (1962) *Totemism*, Harmondsworth: Penguin.

Levy, P. (1984) *The Official Foodies' Handbook*, London: Ebury Press.

—— (1986) *Out to Lunch*, London: Penguin.

Mayle, P. (1990) *A Year in Provence*, London: Pan.

Mennell, S. (1985) *All Manners of Food*, Oxford: Basil Blackwell.

Mintel International (1992) *Eating Out*, London.

Mintz, S. (1985) *Sweetness and Power: The Place of Sugar in History*, Oxford: Basil Blackwell.

Mo, T. (1992) *Sour Sweet*, London: Vintage.

Scaravelli, P. and Cohen, J. (1987) *A Mediterranean Harvest*, Wellingborough: Thorsons.

Smith, D. (1993) *Delia Smith's Summer Collection*, London: BBC Publications.

Tambiah, S.J. (1969) 'Animals are good to think and good to prohibit', *Ethnology* 8, 4: 424–59.

Tannahill, R. (1973) *Food in History*, London: Eyre Methuen.

Wainwright, M. (1991) 'Squatters' rights victory for mites in Stilton cheese', *Guardian*, 4 October.

Young, R. (1989) 'Cod piece', *New Statesman and Society*, 24 November.

Zubaida, S. (1992) 'The social dimensions of Middle Eastern food', in *Culinary Cultures of the Middle East*, Conference Proceedings, London: School of Oriental and African Studies, London.

Chapter 5

Fast food/spoiled identity

Iranian migrants in the British catering trade

Lynn Harbottle

Food, with its primal connotations of nurturance and sustenance, carries powerful psychological, economic, physiological and political meanings. It is also a significant marker of ethnicity (Tremayne 1993) and migrants are frequently very resistant to dietary change. In fact, the maintenance of food habits may serve as a cohesive and stabilising force in a potentially threatening environment (Harbottle 1995: 27–9). The sharing of a food culture is a basis of collective identity and commensality and also a means of expressing both inclusion and otherness (Fischler 1988). For Iranians particularly, the provision of food is a key signifier of acceptance, hospitality and friendship.

Based on ethnographic research conducted amongst dispersed groups of Iranian migrants in England, this chapter explores the characteristics and significance of their food-work in the public sphere. The complex combination of material and symbolic influences propelling these (predominantly male and often well-educated) individuals into the catering trade, are analysed. A recurring and dominant theme in these accounts is of a perceived spoiling of national identity since the Islamic revolution, and it becomes evident that in their work with specific types of non-Iranian food, these migrants seek to disguise and protect their ethnicity.

The data presented here is derived from tape-recorded interviews and informal discussions with about thirty men and two women involved in the catering trade, as well as from participant observations, front- and back-stage, in a number of take-aways and restaurants. Field-work was based in the North-West, Yorkshire and the Midlands, with visits to London, reportedly the centre of the British Iranian community. In writing this account, I have attempted to allow the stories of some of those interviewees[1] to illustrate the diverse forces which have led to individuals taking up employment in what is widely perceived, both by academics and in popular stereotypes, to be a low-status occupation.

ETHNIC MINORITIES AND THE FOOD INDUSTRY

People from a number of different ethnic minority groups have entered the catering trade, in Britain and in other western countries. In the process, they have often contributed to a significant reshaping of local and national cuisines. However, this appears not to be the case with regard to Iranian migrants in England, despite their considerable involvement in this business (Harbottle 1995) and the particular sophistication and symbolic significance of their food culture.

A number of observers have documented the tendency of migrants to seek employment outside the formal economy and have pinpointed their disproportionate representation in the food trade (Watson 1977: 193, Tze Ching 1990: 10). In fact, such has been the scale of ethnic minority involvement in the industry that, by the end of the 1970s, the traditional British institution of fish and chip shops had been almost completely taken over by rural Hong Kong migrants (especially in the Midlands and North-West). In part, the take-over stemmed from the willingness of immigrants to work longer hours, as well as their provision of a much wider menu selection than their competitors (Watson 1977: 194).

However, in these studies it appears that the proprietors were frequently relatively uneducated and rarely spoke English, which meant they had severely limited job prospects within the British labour market. They were clearly distinguished from university graduates of similar origins, who obtained professional jobs and more readily interacted with their British counterparts (Watson 1977: 195). In contrast, the majority of Iranians working in this business appear to be fluent in English and have been educated to at least 'GCE' and 'A'-level standard in this country. Many also hold degrees. Their movement into the industry therefore requires further investigation.

Moreover, Chinese, Indians and others entering the take-away food industry have significantly modified the range of foods available and facilitated the transformation of British tastes (for example, curry is now considered almost as British as roast beef, Fishlock 1994: 25). In so doing they have also contributed to the success of certain ethnic restaurants (Watson 1977: 195, Pong 1986: 5). However, in the case of Iranian entrepreneurs, no such impact is apparent. This is especially noteworthy in view of the highly developed and aesthetically sophisticated nature of Persian[2] cuisine (Shaida 1992).

IRANIAN MIGRANTS AND THE BRITISH LABOUR MARKET

Considerable attention has been paid to the conceptualisation of ethnic minority economic activities (Tze Ching 1990). The terms 'ethnic economy' (originating from middleman minorities literature) and 'ethnic enclave economy' (deriving from labour segmentation theories) are often used interchangeably to designate individual minority employment sectors that coexist with the mainstream economy (Light *et al.* 1994). It is not within the scope of this chapter to review the wider debate, but I have accepted the contention that 'ethnic enclaves', which require spatial clustering and tend to focus on employee income/exploitation, largely overlooking the self-employed, may be encompassed within the more general and wider term 'ethnic economy'. This concept appears more salient to the analysis of Iranian migrants' economic activities, the majority of whom are business owners (Light *et al.* 1994).

It is often assumed that ethnic economies are homogeneous; in reality, sub-groups composed, for example, of different religious affiliations, have been shown to network separately from each other and demonstrate markedly different economic clustering patterns (Light *et al.* 1993). There are no official data available concerning Iranian economic activities in this country.[3] However, in Los Angeles (the largest single centre of Iranian settlement in the USA) Iranian Jews are more likely to engage in the wholesale and retail sales of clothing and jewellery, Armenians in finance, real estate and insurance, Bahais in durable goods manufacture and health and legal services and Shi'ites in the construction industry and durable goods manufacture (Light *et al.* 1993).

In Britain, research on other ethnic groups also indicates regional trends. For example, Manchester was historically the international commercial centre of the textile industry. Recent migrants from Pakistan have, like Jewish immigrants before them, chosen to enter an already well-established clothing trade, carving out a specific niche by supplying cheap clothing which is particularly popular with market-traders (Werbner 1990). This study is specifically concerned with the economic activities of Shi'ite Iranians; although resident in different regions – the North-West, Yorkshire and the Midlands – they demonstrated a high degree of consensus in their explanations of the causal factors resulting in an apparent clustering within the catering trade.

> *Naser*: I know why they all went into take-aways. Most of them, they came to study . . . and then they stopped getting money from [the] government, you know, they couldn't get any more grant[s] . . . so they started working . . . and one of the first guys who really started it all . . . he started a pizza place . . . started to employ these [Iranians]. They all got hard [up] and had to work there. . . . They all learned the trade and realised it's no bother [and] everyone likes [pizza].

A combination of economic, social and political influences are implicated in the movement of Iranians into the food industry. In some respects these are similar to those experienced by other migrants, in particular the difficulty of finding jobs within the mainstream labour market. In addition, the Iranian revolution and subsequent international sequelae have profoundly affected the economic (and social) lives of these migrants.

Initial movement into the catering trade

Prior to the Islamic revolution of 1979, there had been a constant movement of Iranian students to Britain and other western countries. These were mainly young, single and relatively affluent males, the majority intending to return to Iran upon completion of their studies (Gilanshah 1990). However, the flow of government and private funding ceased following the revolution, forcing overseas students to seek temporary work to support themselves. Their political status as temporary residents and need for flexible hours also contributed to their choice of the fast food trade. Reza's story provides an example of the specific and immediate impact of these events. He arrived in Britain in 1976 in his early 20s; limited by the Iranian government's funding policy, he studied mathematics. As he observes:

Reza: [L]ater it wasn't really important what kind of a course you wanted to do – unfortunately – 1978 – we had [the] revolution, so everybody had a feeling for politics, you weren't much concerned with what you were studying or whether you actually studied or not . . . [but] I wanted to carry on . . . [however] it seemed of secondary importance.

Upon graduation in 1981, he had hoped to continue to higher degree level, but, unable to obtain financial support from the new Islamic government in Iran and hit by a massive increase in overseas students' fees in Britain, he was obliged to seek temporary employment. His student visa having expired, he lived, like a number of Iranians at that time, under a constant threat of deportation to what he believed to be a hostile home environment, where 'western indoctrinated' graduates were reportedly being imprisoned. His uncertain political status also restricted his opportunities to work and influenced his decision to enter the food trade.

Reza: At the time I started in '81, I mean, my visa was just about to run out and it was only a visa for studying, it wasn't permanent . . . and didn't allow me to work, so it had to be cash in hand, and usually the easiest kind of job that you find in that situation is catering. . . . Even with English students, the ones who want extra cash . . . they usually end up working in the pubs or restaurants – any kind of catering business. . . . I always hoped I'd do something, take on a job which had something more to do with what I studied . . .

Like many less well-qualified immigrants, he resorted to the informal sector of the labour market. Initially he worked for a few hours a week at an Indian restaurant. Later, he joined a number of his companions serving in a take-away owned by an Iranian friend: 'I only went there when I had decided I wanted to go into the same business. I just went to pick up some ideas.'

Having sought political asylum in 1983, the stress and uncertainty finally ended two years later when he heard that his application had been successful.

Reza: [T]hen I knew: I can either start my own business . . . I had already saved and had some money [to] carry on studying . . . [but I decided] to make a business first and then go back – not knowing that once you dip your head into it, you can't get it out!

He formed a partnership with one of his friends and, having taken over an existing take-away, they initially sold burgers and a few frozen pizzas. As they built up trade and became more experienced, they gradually expanded the menu by adding a range of kebabs. They also improved the quality of the food served, for example by making their own pizzas. Business, which had been slow to begin with, increased steadily.

Their experience seems to be typical of those who entered the trade in the early stages of its development. Prior to the mid-1980s, the demand for fast food grew enormously and there were few outlets, so that it became a highly lucrative proposition (Pong 1986: 4). As a result, in addition to those who entered the catering industry as students or graduates, other Iranians with professional experience also began to drift into it at this time. Their influx was not due solely to the financial 'pull' of the trade, it was also influenced by the decline in the British national economy. Mehdi, for example, had held a job as an electronic engineer but the recession led to the company he worked for going bankrupt. He helped out temporarily in his cousin's take-away and then he and his English wife decided to start their own business.

The emergence of a distinct ethnic economy

In the aftermath of the Islamic revolution and the Iran–Iraq war, increasing numbers of more permanent exiles and refugees arrived in western Europe and North America. Their origins were more heterogeneous in terms of age, marital status, social class, religion, ethnic background and prior western experience (Kamalkhani 1991, Lipson 1992). By this stage, an increasing concentration of Iranians within the take-away business was leading to the development of an ethnic economy, which served to attract new arrivals. For example, Amir was married with one young child when he came to the UK in 1989. He was a political refugee, following imprisonment under the Islamic regime. Members of his wife's family were already settled in the North of England and he spent the first three months living with them as he tried to re-adjust. For the next year and a half, he worked for his brother-in-law in his pizza take-away, then for another fast food venture, before setting up his own business, in 1993. The involvement of other Iranians was influential in his decision-making and reassured him that it was a successful means of providing an income.

Within the developing ethnic economy, bonds of trust, loyalty and credit served to further attract co-ethnics. Amir, like Reza and many other Iranians interviewed, chose to establish a business partnership in the initial stages of his business development. Such joint ventures seem to offer a degree of security if one or both partners are inexperienced or if the premises are situated in an unfamiliar neighbourhood. Generally partners who were Iranian but also well-known, trusted and from the same ethnic and religious background were preferred. For example, both Reza and his partner were Azeri (from the Turkish-speaking area of Azerbaijan) and had known each other for a considerable length of time.

Kinship ties (and occasionally marital bonds as in the case of Mehdi and Fiona) were also good grounds for such a lasting partnership. In some instances Turkish co-owners were chosen, particularly if the Iranian was Azeri; less commonly, agreements with members of other groups such as Pakistanis were mentioned (apparently there are a number of Iranian 'sleeping partners' in the booming Midlands Balti trade). Generally, as is indicated by studies of other minority groups (Watson 1977: 192), the goal appears to be to move towards individual ownership and expansion. Often the capital investment required is obtained predominantly from personal savings and family resources and both Amir and Reza preferred to take the time to accrue personal savings and relied on additional funding from family members in Iran, rather than be heavily indebted to British banks. Within ethnic economies, credit arrangements are also important, particularly in the early stages of business development.

Not only was the autonomy and flexibility of self-employment considered to be preferable to working for someone else, many Iranians had been repelled by the discrimination they had encountered within the formal labour market. In a number of other Iranian migrant communities, those obliged to rely on the mainstream economy also experience occupational and financial disadvantage, such that highly qualified individuals are often obliged to accept relatively unskilled and poorly paid jobs (Pliskin 1987, Kamalkhani 1991, Light *et al.* 1993). At times avoidance of overt racial harassment seems to provide an even stronger incentive to avoid the formal sector. Hence, the catering trade may particularly suit the needs of this and other ethnic minority groups by providing an 'unobtrusive niche on the fringe of the British economy', allowing interaction with the host culture as far as possible on their own terms (Watson 1977: 194).

Amir: You can't get a job here [in the UK] if you're black ... for example we have twenty (Iranian owned) take-aways – eighteen or nineteen owners have got a qualification. . . . I know someone else, [he's] got a job in a company. They gave him a hard time and he left his job and went to [a] take-away.

It is predominantly Iranian men who have taken up work in the take-away food business, but a small number of women, like Floreeda, are also involved. Her account clearly illustrates the impact of discriminatory practices on the movement of Iranians into the ethnic economy. Prior to the revolution, she had been an accountant in a car manufacturing company in Iran but she resigned, in anticipation that female staff would be forced out of work by the Islamic junta, and applied for a visa to visit her brother in Britain. A year later (1985) she arrived and stayed with him for six months. She intended to acquire a British certificate in accountancy but, meanwhile, her brother had opened a take-away and she began to help out. She then realised that even with qualifications she would be unlikely to find a job, in view of the discrimination she perceived towards immigrants: 'I think they prefer English people rather than foreigners, especially when they know you're from the Middle East, it's worse . . . '.

Instead, she invested in her brother's business. Floreeda now owns 25 per cent of the shares and considers herself to work part-time, with an input of 36 hours weekly! This also allows her to undertake further training (as a beauty therapist). When she started college she became deeply disturbed by the attitudes and behaviour of many of the students (mainly young, white, working-class women).

Floreeda: [T]heir attitude towards foreigners is bad . . . they usually look at foreigners like this [demonstrates look of distaste] . . . they don't want to get close to them . . . if there is someone else they won't work with [a] foreigner. . . . You feel awful. . . . They watch you. . . . I hate that.

Her exposure to such discrimination has made her more aware of racism within wider society and she has become increasingly concerned at the apparent upsurge in racial aggression in recent years.

Floreeda: I know a girl, she's Iranian . . . she got a note [through] her door, saying 'Foreigner go home'. . . . I don't feel secure . . . one day they [may] realise . . . I'm the only foreigner in this road . . . [and] set fire to my house or something – what can you do? It wasn't like that five years ago. I notice it more [now] . . . especially in college . . . sometimes when I come home I say: 'Oh my God, I don't want to go back to college again.' . . . That's why I'm glad I've got my own job, I don't need to work for them.

Clearly, Floreeda sees self-employment as a means of protection against discrimination from employers and/or fellow work-mates. Nevertheless, even on their own territory, Iranian entrepreneurs are always vulnerable to the possibility of racial abuse from customers and need to remain vigilant at all times.

Consolidation and diversification

Whereas in the early days of its development the fast food trade was highly lucrative, from the late 1980s onwards market growth has declined slightly whilst the number of outlets has proliferated. Competition has become increasingly fierce, with intense price discounting by the largest chains, resulting in a squeeze on profit margins for all involved (Caines 1994).

The soaring number of outlets has led to geographical diversification, with would-be entrepreneurs now establishing businesses in more peripheral zones (Caines 1994). Traders are also constrained by the consumer-driven market, for example, needing to provide an increasingly diverse menu selection.

Reza: All the time you need to be [working] to keep increased sales going. I mean, probably now is the time to do a new thing – possibly delivery. Usually, once you do something new you pick up some more sales, then after a while it goes a bit steady, then either you introduce something new to improve it again or if you carry along the same line it tends to drop.

Although industrialists optimistically forecast that, with ever-changing consumer tastes and expanding leisure time, the market will not become saturated (Caines 1994), Reza's experience shows that to survive traders need to be highly innovative and adaptive. Even so, success for small businesses is not easily guaranteed.

Having built up their business, Reza and his partner purchased a second shop in 1989. However, a combination of factors, related to the situation of the premises, management difficulties and poor accounting, led to its failure to generate income and the partners eventually had to get rid of it, after making huge losses.

Baqer was even more unfortunate; he too had succeeded in developing a successful business and decided to buy a second outlet. However, this required high-level investment and the new business did not prosper sufficiently to support the interest payments on the loans he had taken out. He went into liquidation and now, in his 50s, he is endeavouring to start again, at a stage when it is acknowledged to be particularly difficult to cope with the long hours and heavy work which the catering business entails.

> *Naser*: Age-wise I think it's affected them as well, [when] they were young they could do several shifts, late nights. They all got, now, so many other commitments, wife, kids, family – they're finding it difficult – they can't work like they used to, so I think that's why they're trying to move into different lines . . .

Others have attempted to diversify into other less strenuous occupations. For example, Yousef has recently opened a gift shop and if it proves profitable, he hopes to sell his take-away. In this study, only one interviewee had succeeded in moving out of the food business altogether. He went back to college and is now working as a dental technician. His view, in common with many others, was that those who had entered the trade prior to the mid-1980s and were now well established would remain successful, but for recent entrants, the prospects are fairly bleak.

> *Naser*: I know a lot of people who have started just recently and they're not doing well at all . . . bankrupt . . . too many of them about now . . . too much competition – Manchester, Sheffield, up North – Newcastle – everywhere. . . . Even other take-aways – there used to be only a few Chinese or fish and chips but getting too many. Some of them I know, they're all moving into different lines. . . . [Others] are established okay but it's not like it was before – a few years ago you'd open a place and guarantee . . . making it.

For many the desire to diversify is countered by the limitations of previous experience and established networks. Hence, Reza, who feels he has lost the opportunity to further his education, sees his choices as restricted to some other role within the food trade. Increasingly, as is typical of other ethnic minority economies (Werbner 1990), businesses have expanded both vertically and horizontally. Larger, highly capitalised firms have emerged at the lower levels of supply, for example wholesaling, and in Newcastle upon Tyne one key Iranian company reportedly dominates the entire British doner kebab meat supply.

Hamid is a distributor for this wholesaler, as well as running his own businesses. He came to Britain only recently (1990) having been active in the import/export trade in Iran. Initially, he had attempted to sell Turkish machine-made carpets, but, although cheaper than Persian handmade rugs, these proved not to be a marketable commodity during the economic recession. Realising that the trade in foodstuffs was comparatively stable, Hamid started supplying frozen chips, taking on the sole agency for a Dutch company in 1991. He then intended to open a food cash-and-carry, believing he could attract enough custom from both Iranian and Turkish fast food and restaurant owners to ensure success. However, he was offered a partnership in a burger chain owned by a Canadian immigrant and recognised this to be a more secure proposition; it has since proved highly successful. Hamid has continually diversified and expanded his interests; he still distributes doner kebab meat, as well as overseeing his import company. In addition to chips, he now also imports tomato paste, 'pizza cheese', pepperoni and a particular type of sausage made to the burger company's own specifications. He intends to become increasingly self-reliant in future, for example by establishing his own burger factory.

IRANIAN INVISIBILITY WITHIN THE CATERING TRADE

Ethnic entrepreneurs within the fast food business have commonly modified take-away menus in distinctive ways. In Germany, Turkish entrepreneurs have successfully created a market niche for doner kebab such that it has become symbolic of Turkish identity. Additionally, by applying English language names like 'Mckebap', which evoke associations with powerful multinational food companies, they have also been able to manipulate the meanings of the kebab and, in the process, have to some extent transformed the stereotypes of Turkish migrants (Caglar 1993).

Seen in this context, it appears particularly striking that, despite their large-scale involvement in the British take-away food trade, the Iranian impact has been negligible (by comparison with, for example, the marked influence of Chinese food in this country). This is in spite of the view expressed by many of the Iranians interviewed that the British lack a distinguishable or developed cuisine of their own.

> *Mehdi*: English people don't have a food culture as such, they eat any food so long as it is hot but they don't know anything about it.

> *Floreeda*: I've heard that most Iranians [in the USA] are dealing with cars or petrol stations . . . but here it's a cold country, food is [the] best thing . . . [and] English people haven't got different types of food . . . just fish and chips.

The few proprietors who had tried to market Persian dishes reported that the taste had been too subtle for the undiscerning British palate. In most take-aways a combination of burgers, kebabs and pizzas were sold; some specialised only in pizzas. These were thought to be popular chiefly because they provided a vehicle for the consumption of chilli sauce, with hot chilli pizza being a particular favourite of customers! Interestingly, kebabs, identified generically as an Iranian food by proprietors, were sold in the awareness that the general British public consider them to be of Turkish/Mediterranean origin.

Food is a powerful marker of ethnicity and to allow one's food to be rejected or treated with contempt[4] is also to face possible self-humiliation. By serving non-Iranian food, these entrepreneurs have been able to protect, as well as disguise, their ethnicity. Not only does the food served – ubiquitous, relatively bland and global – give no indication as to the ethnic affiliation of the owner, even the names of many of the take-aways act to further disguise their identities. Many such names conjure up Italian-American imagery, for example 'The Godfather', while others simply designate the fact that pizza or other food items are available. Sometimes proprietors admitted the need to use dissimulation and pretence in order to protect their identities.

> *Floreeda*: [W]hen I'm working, I'm not telling them this place belongs to Iranians, I'm telling them I'm Italian or half Greek/ half Italian something, because I'm scared one day they'll break

everything.... Before [the] revolution I've heard that [to be] Iranian was [considered] very good, because they thought we [were] really posh, lots of money [and] oil but after [the] revolution [it changed]. I can't tell them when I'm working I'm Iranian.... Once it happened ... I was serving a customer – daytime – and he said ... 'What nationality have you got?' ... I said 'I'm half Greek' and then he said 'I've heard that, a friend of mine told me, that bloke in here is Iranian.' I said 'No ... we are Greek, we are not Iranian in here.' That customer, he was with a tattoo and rough ... he said, 'Good, good, you are not Iranian' ... that's why I have to keep quiet!

Her account highlights a perceived transformation and spoiling of Iranian national identity since the revolution. It also demonstrates the fact that all ethnic minority groups are not equally subject to discrimination. This is underlined by research in the USA among both black and white undergraduates, which indicates that Iranians are considered the least desirable ethnic group with which to interact as friends, neighbours or in the workplace (Sparrow and Chretien 1993). Other studies in the USA also suggest that they are the most shunned and misunderstood of all immigrant groups (Hoffman 1990). Most of those interviewed felt that to admit to being Iranian was to play on negative public perceptions and stereotypes, particularly of Islamic fundamentalism, and therefore to incur hostile reactions. The response of many of these individuals was to attempt to disguise their ethnicity and to pass as more acceptable others, such as Italians, Greeks or Turks.[5]

The invisibility of Iranian cuisine is also reflected in the restaurant sector. In fact, the only apparent exception is demonstrated, not by those serving food to the public, but by the backstage food suppliers; some of these select names which openly advertise their nationality, presumably to enlist the interests of Iranian customers from a range of ethnic and religious backgrounds. Despite the rapid growth in popularity of 'ethnic' restaurants generally (Miller 1994: 19, 1995: 3), and the fact that Iranian cuisine is highly elaborated, there appear to be few such outlets in this country. A common perception amongst Iranian entrepreneurs was that these had lost popularity since the early 1980s for a number of reasons.

Mehdi: A lot of people haven't heard of Iran and there's Islamic prejudice. If I call it an Iranian restaurant, how many people am I going to get? Like when England plays Italy at football and loses, all the pizza places will be attacked!

Fiona: If the revolution hadn't happened, Iran would have been a main holiday destination like Turkey now is.

Floreeda: I don't think a restaurant is good [here], especially Persian food, because [British people] don't know about Persian food.

Increasingly, global influences, such as international tourism, migration, communication and trade links, serve to shape a 'national cuisine' and determine its popularity. In the West, those who have travelled abroad on holiday or read cookery books increasingly seek out authentic and exotic national cuisines (Zubaida 1994: 44–5) and 'ethnic' restaurants run by migrant communities have been obliged to respond to this search. Many interviewees felt the impact of the Islamic revolution to be particularly significant, first in creating negative stereotypes about Iranians which were believed to deter the British from trying their food, and second through the paralysis of tourism within Iran and consequent lack of exposure of outsiders to the food culture; this was contrasted by interviewees with the popularity of cuisines from tourist haunts such as Greece and Turkey.

Additionally, whereas some groups, such as Indians, were thought to have large enough local communities to provide patronage for their own restaurants, the Iranian population, especially in the Midlands and the North, was considered too small to provide adequate support for a distinctively ethnic restaurant. The high level of initial investment required was also considered to be detrimental, particularly in an uncertain economic climate.

Amir: After [the] recession Iranians didn't take a risk to open a restaurant because so many restaurants went bankrupt. That's why we stick with fast food. . . . I could take a risk with Italian food – people in England know Italian food but they don't know Iranian food.

However, some informants reported that Iranian restaurants are still flourishing in Manchester and London, where the Iranian population is larger and the people are considered to be more cosmopolitan and open to new tastes.

Naser: I've had friends who started restaurants with Iranian food, some of them are doing OK, you know, it depends which area and what part, I mean some in Manchester [are] quite good ... and there's some in London, quite a lot and they do quite well, I mean they even get customers apart from Iranians!

Upon enquiry, the majority of such restaurants supposedly existing in Manchester appeared to have gone out of business, although there is one which seems to be doing well. The whole family are involved in the running of this enterprise. They outlined other problems specific to Iranian would-be restaurateurs; one major obstacle appears to be the lack of skilled chefs here, owing to the security of their occupational status in Iran.

Azam: [I]t is very difficult to run a Persian restaurant and you have to have a chef, a qualified chef and we don't have any. . . . [And the] food we buy – the meat is very, very expensive. And when we go to a Persian restaurant the main thing is [the] meat and it has to be good. . . . We have to pay a lot of money to buy fillet of lamb.

Like many others interviewed, Azam elects to apply the label 'Persian', with its connotations of former empire and pre-Islam, rather than using the more negatively perceived 'Iranian' identity. She stressed the high quality demanded in the preparation of Persian food and precedence given to the place of meat within the meal, emphasising the fact that, unlike other food cultures, there could be no cheap alternatives. Nor could there be any simple shortcuts to the intensive preparation required and she felt that the demanding nature of the job, in terms of time input and working conditions, was a powerful disincentive to entering the trade.

Azam: [I]t's very difficult – the person who cooks, like my husband; he spends most of his time in the kitchen. While he's cooking kebab, he's facing the big huge barbecue and it's very, very hot. You cannot stand it . . . most all of them are men. . . . [A]ll of us – four of us – we work really hard, we don't have any social life. My husband, sometimes he comes here and goes to [the] kitchen at 7 am and doesn't leave until 10–11 pm . . . this is our life.

Prior to migration to Britain in 1975, Azam's husband had owned a chain of kebab restaurants in Iran. Once settled in

Manchester, Azam became increasingly bored with her domestic role and she and her husband decided to re-enter the catering trade together. They have now established a reputation among Iranians in the North and their current enterprise (designated a 'Persian-Mediterranean' restaurant, and opened in 1993) has attracted a loyal following, not only from the region but even drawing visitors from as far away as Scotland.

> *Azam*: As soon as we opened, a lot of Iranians heard, and these were people who had been coming to our restaurants and following us whenever we opened a restaurant. Very nice people – classy people, I call them – very easy to work with. ... [W]e never had [a] problem struggling, thanks to all our Iranian customers who [have] been following us and supporting us.

RESTAURANTS AND THE TRANSFORMATION OF FOOD CULTURES

The success of certain ethnic restaurants is related to the ways in which they have been able to enlist the interests of a specific sector of the population. For example, Thai cuisine has enjoyed a recent growth in popularity. Through observations and discussions with staff in a number of Thai restaurants it seems that several factors have contributed to their relative success. Increasing media coverage, and especially television programmes focusing on Thai cookery, and the impact of tourism and travel programmes have created a general receptiveness towards this cuisine. Additionally, taste and aesthetic resonances with Chinese and Indian foods apparently attract people already familiar with local versions of those food cultures.

In one Thai restaurant, the manager reported that, apart from the high quality of the food, the aspect most positively lauded was the degree of deference demonstrated towards customers by the (largely female and exotically clad) staff. In this case, the enrolment of British interests may also involve a manipulation of customers' fantasies regarding power and sexuality and specifically of a subordinate and sexually available female other.

Sociological studies of McDonald's indicate that it enjoys worldwide success precisely because it has a theory concerning the interests of its customers and it attempts to play upon their dreams and fantasies in order to increase sales (Law 1984: 187). Hence, it 'stages its dramas' in ways that appear attractive to as many potential customers as possible: for example, in the light of the current concern for a 'healthy' diet the nutrient composition of food items is advertised; in order to attract the interest of children (and through them to reach their parents) a number of appealing activities, characters and toys are provided.

Throughout history, a number of 'invading' cuisines have been modified, and often changed beyond recognition, in response to local demand (Mars 1983). Entrepreneurs from a number of ethnic groups have learned that in order to succeed in the British market, some degree of adaptation – if not total transformation – is required (Tapper and Zubaida 1994: 13), although, as the up-market sector of the tourist trade expands, the demand for more 'authentic' dishes increases. The Chinese food consumed in Britain has been recorded as bearing little relation to any 'authentic' Chinese dishes (Pong 1986: 5); similarly, the current craze for Balti meals has sparked heated debates over the origins of this segment of the Asian catering trade (Tredre 1995). Italian restaurants, too, may be more accurately described as 'English restaurants with an Italian style'; long menus tend to replace the smaller selection offered by restaurateurs in Italy, fresh fruit has vanished and the sauces are made thicker to satisfy British preferences (Mars 1983).

So far it seems that Iranian restaurateurs have been less successful in their attempts to establish a significant niche in the market and to enlist the interests of non-Iranian clients. This appears to be partly due to differences in Iranian and British food combinations, aesthetic and textural preferences and other direct, food-related factors as well as to wider marketing strategies. For example, although Azam reflected positively on the success of her restaurant with Iranians, she was aware of the need to attract other customers, yet experienced some ambivalence towards the idea, perhaps fearing their needs would clash with the requirements of the established Iranian clientele.

Azam: I can say [the customers are] 95 per cent Iranian. . . . I wish we could get more students – hopefully we will, but right now the number of students is low. . . . What we call . . . special is different to what [British] people are used to. People think it's a 3 course meal, which it's not. We [are] selling 2 of the most popular dishes on the menu . . . a combination of fillet of lamb kebab and mince kebab and rice for £4.50 and the other [special] is whole spring chicken in pieces, flavoured in saffron . . . for £4.50 with rice . . . but I've experienced a couple of non-Iranian people [who] came here and . . . when I explained to them they were surprised [that] there is no starter and no sweet . . .

Azam is aware that if her family intends to sell Persian cuisine to a British market, they will need to be prepared to make some adaptations and in particular to cater to the British sweet tooth.

Azam: We are going to advertise for students. . . . We're planning to change the menu . . . and hopefully after that we can advertise [in] more places. . . . I feel we have so many kebabs and rice and I find that a little dry for our non-Iranian customers, so we'd like to add [a] few more *khoreshes* – casseroles. . . . The sweets, I'm not very proud of the ones we serve . . . we're not the type of people who are interested in having dessert; you know, back at home we used to have melon and fruit.

During one visit to this restaurant, with an English friend, I also noted a discordance between my representation of Persian cuisine, based on home dining, and the meal served (Harbottle 1995). To outsiders, the sight of the unadorned main dish, without the customary extras, such as *torchi* and salad, appeared bare and uninspiring. When dining there with Iranians, I had, it appears, been able to apply symbolic value to the meal, but this aesthetic exercise was not possible with a non-initiand, and as a result, the previous ambience proved elusive on this occasion.

A restaurant may be thought of as a stage upon which individuals act out particular roles. Consideration of the setting and decor provides the first step in understanding how customers choose (or avoid) a particular venue and why they behave in distinctive ways within it (Shelton 1990). Intrigued by the descriptions, provided by provincial interviewees, of a thriving Iranian restaurant trade in London, I visited Kensington and ate lunch in the first such establishment I found. From the exterior, the name evoked images of a glorious Persian empire, whilst the premises themselves looked in need of a coat of paint. As in the case of other restaurants in this trendy up-market area of London, a minimum cover charge of £10 was set. Inside, the atmosphere was subdued and fusty, with a slight air of seediness. The lighting was dim, a worn carpet covered the floor and on the walls only a single frieze was identifiably Iranian; British light music played in the background. The waiter reported business to be slow and there were only six other diners during my visit – two ageing Aquinas scholars, and two middle-aged couples, one Iranian and the other a British/ Iranian pair.

The chef informed me he had been recruited in Iran twenty-five years ago to work in this restaurant. At that time it had been a thriving establishment, predominantly owing to large numbers of Iranian tourists flooding into London; contrary to the accounts given by provincial interviewees, there have never been many British customers. Since the revolution, the number of Iranian travellers has declined and the business is now struggling. According to this chef, few Iranian owners have the marketing expertise to attract the British.

Advertising can only work if the message latches on to something which the consumer perceives to be desirable. In the case of this and other Iranian restaurants I visited briefly, it seemed that the owners weren't quite sure whose interest they were trying to attract, or which sector of the market they were aiming at. For example, a meal in this restaurant was not much cheaper than in a Lebanese enterprise resembling 'a grand European hotel on the colonial fringe' (Shelton 1990) with its plate glass frontage, parlour palms, immaculately clad waiters and lyrical menu. Nor could it compete with some of the cheaper cafe bars, which successfully targeted young trendy middle-class employees, who wanted a 'healthy' and quick meal.

It seems that Iranians are generally unclear about how they wish to construct their image and play upon British tastes. This may be due, in part, to the lack of an established restaurant culture in Iran, which dates back only as far as the early twentieth century (Fragner 1994: 66). However, I propose that it is also related to the discrimination Iranian migrants perceive and to a post-revolutionary sense of spoiled identity, which leaves them unable to discern any positive interests within the ethnic majority upon which to draw.

Loss of a national identity

During the reign of the late Shah, a clear movement towards defining a national identity, involving a 'persification' of the language (Tapper 1989: 237), and glorification of pre-Islamic civilisation and empire, took place. This national construction was also shaped by the strong influence of western politics and culture in Iran at that time. Although resisted by many Iranians, it proved attractive in the USA and Europe, leading to stereotypes of a sophisticated, intelligent and wealthy people. This notion of Persian culture is still represented within some circles and is reflected in recent culinary literature:

> [Iran] is a distant land, remote and mysterious; a land of ancient culture and often elegant ritual. It is also a land of remarkably good food . . . many of its dishes can be traced back a thousand years. . . . When the Persians first conquered the ancient world . . . not the least influence was the introduction of their food. . . . To [the Greeks], used to plain fare spiced with little more than hexameters, the sophisticated eating habits of the Persians proved fascinating and sometimes irresistible. . . . Even Herodotus . . . commended the remarkable skills of the Persian bakers and cooks. . . . Indeed, the Persians thought the Greeks remained hungry much of the time because of the dreariness of their food.
>
> (Shaida 1992: 2–3)

Cookery books are especially important in helping to create a national culture and cuisine, and, as Fragner notes, may 'tell us more about a people's collective imagination, symbolic values, dreams and expectations than about actual culinary conditions' (1994: 71). Shaida's book, *The Legendary Cuisine of Persia* (written by an English woman married to an Iranian) promotes a pre-Islamic national construction by evoking an authenticity and superiority of Persian cooking from ancient times; she claims much of the Middle Eastern and Asian repertoire to be of Persian origin. The exoticised notions of culture and cuisine upon which she draws are appealing to European tastes, yet Iranians in the catering trade seem generally unwilling to adopt and extend these images.

Since the Islamic revolution there has been a major uprooting of former constructions of 'nation' and a metamorphosis of identity of Iranians worldwide. For many this has resulted in confusion and a sense of loss. 'Because we have lost our identity . . . we seem a sort of bewildered people. . . . Some people think like that. They have lost their identity, they don't know where they are . . .' (Mostafa). Ironically, it is precisely those who sought refuge or exile away from the Khomeini administration who now find themselves most powerfully stigmatised by the current wave of Islamophobia.

Goffman (1968) first considered the stigma associated with certain marginal groups, including the disabled and some ethnic minorities. Murphy also observes the power of imposed stereotypes, fears and misunderstandings, and the constant battle of those who experience the despoilment of their identities to maintain a sense of self-worth by adopting defensive strategies such as social retreat (1987: 113–22). Dorman (1979) also highlights the role of the media in shaping international stereotypes of Iranians subsequent to the Islamic revolution.

> *Zahra*: Probably that's the reason I feel I can't mix up with them [English] you know. . . . When you're talking about Iran . . . they always say: 'Oh that horrible Khomeini and all this terrorism' . . . but you can't – I can't – keep explaining [to] people what we're like . . .

There seems to be a significant level of internal confusion among exiles and refugees over how to reconstruct Iranian national identity, which is apparently reflected in the catering trade. A restaurant should not be a static object but a process, drawing upon changing societal elements, but in the case of some of the London establishments an ambience of shabbiness and sense of stasis give the impression of a paralysed culture, unsure how to move forward. Accounts given by provincial Iranians of a thriving London scene, with Kensington at its heart, also appear to represent nostalgic memories and conflict with tangible local fragmentation.

We choose to eat out in establishments with others who apparently share our values and thereby mark our cultural boundaries (Finkelstein 1989: 26–7). With so many different ethnic, political and religious interest groups represented amongst Iranians in Britain, it is unsurprising that there is a high degree of mutual mistrust such that the event of dining in the same place could provoke intense anxiety and discomfort. For restaurant owners, this raises the dilemma of whether to broadcast their own affiliations, so restricting their market potential (and leaving themselves personally exposed and vulnerable), or to endeavour to accommodate all interests, under the uniting notion of a 'national culture', as has been attempted in Manchester.

CONCLUSION

The preceding account has illustrated the multiple and intersecting factors which have led to the emergence and consolidation of a distinct Shi'ite Iranian ethnic economy in England, paradoxically based on non-Iranian take-away foods. Both material and symbolic factors have been influential. In particular, discrimination within the formal labour market and nationwide economic decline served as key 'push' factors propelling the movement of these migrants into the informal sector, whilst the autonomy and marginality of take-aways (as well as their profitability) proved highly attractive to migrants struggling with problems of national identity. Although competition within the trade has increased over time and arduous working conditions are a powerful disincentive, nevertheless the take-away business still provides a feasible prospect in a generally gloomy economy.

The immediate political and economic impact of the Islamic revolution was clearly a major influence in precipitating the initial drift into this business. Moreover, the ongoing reverberations, through time and space, of this uprising have continued to resound in the lives of Iranian exiles. Notions of a unified 'Persian' identity, formerly popular in the West, have latterly been undermined by potent Islamophobia and racism, resulting in a strong sense of stigmatisation amongst these migrants. Through the relative invisibility of Iranian cuisine and the need, perceived by proprietors, for ethnic 'passing',[6] the British catering sector reflects not only the current sense of internal cultural fragmentation, in the absence of a tenable unifying national force, but also the power of imposed stereotypes.

NOTES

1 Pseudonyms have been used throughout.
2 That is, its origins pre-date the territorial designation of Iran.
3 Like other Middle Eastern populations, they are categorised under the 'Asian' ethnic grouping for such analysis (OPCS, personal communication).
4 Especially in Iranian culture where it plays a vital part in daily interaction (Harbottle 1995: 27).
5 Such is the comparative familiarity of Greek, Italian and other European foods that these are no longer defined as 'ethnic', according to recent food industry reports (Miller 1986).
6 Muslim Pakistani and Bangladeshi entrepreneurs also manipulate their

ethnicity by marketing their food as 'Indian' and often adopt names which evoke images of Raj and Empire like 'Passage to India', to attract custom.

REFERENCES

Caglar, A. (1993) 'McKebap: doner kebap and Turkish identity in Berlin', Paper given at the Fourth Conference on Research in Consumption, 'Global and the Local Consumption and European Identity', Amsterdam, 8–11 September.

Caines, R. (ed.) (1994) *Fast Food and Home Delivery Outlets, Keynote Reports: An Industry Sector Overview*, 11th edn, London: Keynote Publications.

Dorman, W.A. (1979) 'Iranian people v. US news media: a case of libel', *Race and Class* 1: 57–66.

Finkelstein, J. (1989) *Dining Out: A Sociology of Modern Manners*, Cambridge: Polity Press.

Fischler, C. (1988) 'Food, self and identity', *Social Science Information* 27, 2: 275–92.

Fishlock, T. (1994) 'Hot Spots', *The Telegraph Magazine*, 23 July.

Fragner, B. (1994) 'Social reality and culinary fiction: the perspective of cookbooks from Iran and Central Asia', Chapter 4 in S. Zubaida and R. Tapper (eds) *Culinary Cultures of the Middle East*, London: I.B. Tauris.

Gilanshah, F. (1990) 'The formation of Iranian community in the twin cities, 1983–89', *Wisconsin Sociologist* 27, 4: 11–17.

Goffman, E. (1968) *Stigma: Notes on the Management of Spoiled Identity*, Harmondsworth: Penguin.

Harbottle, L. (1995) '"Palship", parties and pilgrimage: kinship, community formation and self-transformation of Iranian migrants to Britain', *Working Paper No. 9: Representations of Places and Identities*, Keele: Keele University Press.

Hoffman, D.M. (1990) 'Beyond conflict: culture, self and intercultural learning among Iranians in the US', *International Journal of Intercultural Relations* 14, 3: 275–99.

Kamalkhani, Z. (1991) 'Iranians in Norway: adaptation and community formation', *Migration World Magazine* 19, 2: 8–12.

Law, J. (1984) 'How much of society can the sociologist digest at one sitting? The "macro" and the "micro" revisited for the case of fast food', *Studies in Symbolic Interaction* 5: 171–96.

Light, I., Sabagh, G., Bozormehr, M. and Der-Martirosian, C. (1993) 'Internal ethnicity in the ethnic economy', *Ethnic and Racial Studies* 16, 4: 581–97.

—— (1994) 'Beyond the ethnic enclave economy', *Social Problems* 41, 1: 65–80.

Lipson, J.G. (1992) 'The health and adjustment of Iranian immigrants', *Western Journal of Nursing Research* 14, 1: 10–29.

Mars, V. (1983) 'Spaghetti – but not on toast! Italian food in London', in

V. Mars (ed.) *Food in Motion. The Migration of Foodstuffs and Cookery Techniques, The Oxford Symposium Volume 1*, Totnes: Prospect Books.

Miller, S. (ed.) (1986) *Ethnic Foods: UK Catering Market, Industry Trends and Forecasts, Keynote Market Review*, 2nd edn, London: Keynote Publications.

—— (ed.) (1994) *Restaurants: UK Catering Market, Industry Trends and Forecasts, Keynote Market Review*, 7th edn, London: Keynote Publications.

—— (1995) *Ethnic Foods: UK Catering Market Industry Review*, Keynote Market Review, 6th edn, London: Keynote Publications.

Murphy, R. (1987) *The Body Silent*, New York: Henry Holt and Co.

Pliskin, K.L. (1987) *Silent Boundaries: Cultural Constraints on Sickness and Diagnosis of Iranians in Israel*, New Haven: Yale University Press.

Pong, N.N. (1986) 'An empirical study of attitudes towards a Chinese restaurant in Sheffield', unpublished Masters Dissertation, Sheffield University.

Shaida, M. (1992) *The Legendary Cuisine of Persia*, Henley on Thames: Lieuse Books.

Shelton, A. (1990) 'A theatre for eating, looking and thinking: the restaurant as symbolic space', *Sociological Spectrum* 10, 4: 507–26.

Sparrow, K.H. and Chretien, D.M. (1993) 'The social distance perceptions of racial and ethnic groups by college students: a research note', *Sociological Spectrum* 13: 277–88.

Tapper, R. and Zubaida, S. (1994) 'Introduction' to S. Zubaida and R. Tapper (eds) *Culinary Cultures of the Middle East*, London: I.B. Tauris.

Tredre, R. (1995) 'Pukka masters of Balti cast their chilly gaze south', *Observer* 7 May.

Tremayne, S. (1993) 'We Chinese eat a lot: food as a symbol of ethnic identity in Kuala Lumpur', in G. Mars and V. Mars (eds) *Food, Culture and History*, Vol. 1, London: The London Food Seminar.

Tze Ching, L. (1990) 'Ethnic enterprise in the Kansas City metropolitan area: the Chinese', unpublished PhD Thesis, Kansas University.

Watson, J.L. (1977) 'The Chinese: Hong Kong villagers in the British catering trade', Chapter 7 in J.L. Watson (ed.) *Between Two Cultures*, Oxford: Basil Blackwell.

Werbner, P. (1990) 'Renewing an industrial past: British Pakistani enterprises in Manchester', *Migration* 8: 7–41.

Zubaida, S. (1994) 'National, communal and global dimensions in Middle Eastern food cultures', Chapter 2 in S. Zubaida and R. Tapper (eds) *Culinary Cultures of the Middle East*, London: I.B. Tauris.

Chapter 6

'Bacon sandwiches got the better of me'

Meat-eating and vegetarianism in South-East London

Anna Willetts

The saying, 'You are what you eat', is familiar to us all. While rather hackneyed, the frequency with which it is encountered within the social science of food is testimony to the importance of an approach it has come to represent. Food choice is seen as an integral expression of who we are and what we believe in. Here, apparently mundane aspects of food choice are thought to symbolise not only identity on a personal level, but also culturally defined value systems.

Based on research conducted in a South-East London borough this paper will approach the question of identity through an examination of meat-eating and vegetarianism. Vegetarianism is not only a dietary change associated with health, it is also thought to *say something* about the world-views of those who practise it. What I shall argue is that we need, first, to re-appraise what we mean by vegetarianism and, second, to deconstruct the model that positions meat-eating and vegetarianism as oppositional.

In recent years, social scientists eager to unravel the hidden meanings inscribed in food choice have looked to vegetarianism. Their concern reflects the increasing popularity of a vegetarian diet in Britain; 4.5 per cent of the adult population are now vegetarian, more than twice the number of a decade ago (*The Realeat Survey* 1995). It also indicates interest in the process through which individuals *become* vegetarian. Vegetarianism in the West is seldom the diet of a life-long practitioner. Instead, it is usually that of a 'convert', someone who has 'subjected more traditional foodways to critical scrutiny and has subsequently made a deliberate decision to change their eating habits' (Beardsworth and Keil 1992: 253). Academic interest in vegetarianism, therefore, is based primarily on the assumption that its adherents have undergone an explicit process of reflection and have chosen to subscribe to an alternative ideology, one at odds with that of 'the dominant culture' (Twigg 1983: 21).

In analysing vegetarianism then, many social scientists have shared the assumption that meat-eating and vegetarianism are representative of two unique and oppositional world-views (Twigg 1979, 1983, Adams 1990, Fiddes 1992, Spencer 1994, Cox 1994). The apparent barbarity and domination inherent in meat-eating is juxtaposed to the gentle humanity of vegetarianism, and each dietary practice is seen to represent an opposing conceptualisation of the relationship between humans and the natural world.

Before discussing the research I undertook in South-East London, I want to examine briefly the work of three authors who have taken such a 'world-view' perspective.

In one of the first accounts of contemporary western vege-tarianism, the sociologist Julia Twigg argues that within the 'dominant culture', there exists a hierarchy of foods in which red meat is the most highly prized form of nutrition, maintaining a supreme position above the lower-status foods such as white meat, fish, dairy products and fruits and vegetables. Red meat is ascendant because, unlike the other foods, it harnesses the symbolic power of blood. As such, red meat is imbued with vitality, strength and passion and becomes the food of the elites and particularly of men (Twigg 1979, 1983). As we feed upon meat then it becomes the primal way through which we ingest – and suppress – nature.

Twigg suggests, however, that vegetarianism re-evaluates the perceptions of meat found in 'dominant culture'. In choosing to eat down the hierarchy of foods away from red meat, positive associations are inverted. Rather than standing for maleness in an approved sense, meat 'is seen as a false, macho stereotype of masculinity. Thus "strength" and "power" become "cruelty" and "aggression"; masculine vigour and courage become violence and the forces of human destructiveness' (1983: 27). An additional factor in this inversion is the symbolic dissociation of meat from life-giving qualities. Thus, while meat is 'dead' food, symbolic of decay at both a physical and moral level, vegetarian food is reconceptualised as pure and full of 'the essence of life' (Twigg 1983: 28). Vegetarianism, then, not unlike the health food and wholefood movements, promises devotees a this-worldly salvation (Atkinson 1980, 1983, Dubisch 1985). Only through vegetarianism can we return to a 'natural empathy' with animals and the wider environment around us (Twigg 1983: 28).

Carol Adams also proposes a quintessential relationship between men and meat. In a polemical and emotive account entitled *The Sexual Politics of Meat* (1990), she suggests that meat-eating is a symbol of patriarchy. 'Meat-eating', she says, 'is the re-inscription of male power at every meal' (1990: 187). For Adams, the fate of women and animals is inextricably linked. They are both tyrannised and violated by men and her analysis equates the physical and sexual subjugation of women to the butchery of animals. Thus, feminism and vegetarianism are similar struggles against a common – male – oppressor.

Adams's account – essentially a textual analysis – roams freely through time and culture. She delights in making bold statements and, even when confined to food practices in the West, her argument suffers badly from over-stretched analogies between men and meat that give rise to misplaced assertions. At one point she even argues that, 'just as it is thought a woman cannot make it on her own, so we think that vegetables cannot make a meal on their own' (1990: 33). Leaving objectivism aside she champions the vegetarian cause and urges the reader to stop eating meat because only through removing meat from a meal can the structure of patriarchal culture be actively threatened.

Finally, in a more recent account of meat-eating as a 'natural symbol', Nick Fiddes argues that the high value placed on meat is contingent upon its symbolic importance, 'as a tangible representation of human control of, and superiority over, nature' (1991: 6). Unlike Adams he does not argue that we constantly exult in our domination of animals with every mouthful of meat. Rather, the principle of 'power over nature' is an omnipresent thread running through 'our' culture and 'carnivoracity' is simply the primary vehicle through which this can be demonstrated (1991: 3).

For Fiddes, then, the increasing popularity of vegetarianism provides evidence of fundamental developments in society. In tandem with the growing concern for green issues, vegetarianism offers a direct challenge to this prevailing ethos of environmental domination. As he concludes:

Since 'carnivoracity' has long been a Natural Symbol by which we have expressed our society's quest for dominance, the food's diminishing status could well be symptomatic of the wane of outdated ideals. If so, the turbulently declining reputation of meat, at the advent of the third millennium, may be a harbinger of the evolution of new values.

(Fiddes 1991: 233)

For all three authors, then, meat-eating – the literal incorporation of the animal – is read as the ultimate expression of domination, both of women and of the natural world. In contrast, vegetarianism is seen to valorise a biocentric attitude to the environment in which humans live in harmony with each other and with the natural world around them.

Meat-eating and vegetarianism are thus portrayed as two distinct dietary practices in Britain, each accompanied by its own unique world-view. My own research in South-East London, however, does not support this conclusion because the latter applies a universal meaning to meat that does not stand up to scrutiny. Importantly, my evidence suggests that meat-eating and vegetarianism are not as different as is often suggested. In many instances it is impossible to see a clear distinction between the diets of the two groups. Furthermore, rather than holding exclusive sets of beliefs, meat-eaters and vegetarians share many similar views on health, animal rights, factory farming and environmental issues.

Such a reappraisal of the meaning of meat was also undertaken by Brian Morris in his account of meat-eating in southern Malawi. He too is critical of the trend to generalise meanings, arguing that 'to universalise vegetarian sentiments is hardly conducive to cross-cultural understanding' (1994: 20). I would perhaps take this further and argue that generalisations, though useful analytical devices, all too often fail to account for everyday practice.

Indeed, I want to stress that the vegetarians who participated in this study were not always more environmentally aware than non-vegetarians. In certain circumstances eating meat was also one outcome of a respect for nature and, for one environmental group in South-East London, was the culmination of a life lived in symbiosis with the environment. In an apparent rewriting of the Enlightenment principle of 'power over nature' eating meat can be the ultimate acknowledgement of the power of nature.

THE RESEARCH LOCATION

This article is based on field-work conducted in a South-East London borough during 1993–4 (see Keane and Willetts 1996,

Caplan *et al.* 1997). The borough covers an area of 13.7 square miles and has a population of just over a quarter of a million. Within the borough there are a number of different areas, each with their own character and history. However, a broad division can be seen between the relatively poor areas to the north and the more affluent areas to the south. Unemployment, for example, is highest in the north (24 per cent compared to 17 per cent in the borough as a whole). The north also has a higher proportion of council tenants, residents from social class D and E and one-parent families. Of the residents in the north, 38 per cent are from minority ethnic groups. The south is more suburban in character, however pockets of poverty do exist (Hyde *et al.* 1989).

Empirical data was gathered through a range of techniques including semi-structured interviews, participant observation, food diaries and food frequency questionnaires. In total, 158 people were interviewed in depth, comprised of 134 local residents and twenty-four professionals including doctors, dieticians, cookery teachers, community workers and retailers working in the borough. Interviews lasted up to three hours and second interviews were also conducted. The interview format was designed to be flexible, allowing participants to discuss their concerns on a broad range of topics from shopping and expenditure, food preparation and consumption, health and healthy eating, diet and body image, to vegetarianism and food production and processing. Participant observation was conducted in a range of settings including slimming clubs, cookery classes, health workshops, schools, community groups and environmental pressure groups.

WHAT IS A VEGETARIAN?

I want to begin by asking the question: 'What is a vegetarian?' Of the 134 local residents, nineteen identified themselves as 'vegetarian' and four as 'vegan', together representing 17 per cent of the resident sample. The majority were also female (sixteen) and middle class (nineteen) and young (20–39 years old as compared to 20–87 years old for the residents as a whole). They had 'converted' to their particular dietary regime between two to eighteen years ago. Thirteen other participants also defined themselves as 'ex-vegetarian'.

In nutritional terms, the categories of vegetarian and vegan covered a varied set of dietary practices. Self-defined vegetarians did not confine themselves to a meat-free diet, but ate a wide range of meats, most commonly chicken and fish, but also pork and beef. One 'vegan' also ate bacon and another ate fish. In fact, only eight of the vegetarians in the study did not eat any meat. While acknowledging that the sample was relatively small, the fact that 66 per cent of the self-defined vegetarians incorporated meat into their diet should not go unnoticed.

For some vegetarians and vegans eating meat appeared as a momentary 'lapse' in an otherwise unblemished career, and consequently did not impinge on their identity as vegetarian. This lapse could be prompted by several factors. For some people it was the desire not to appear impolite when given meat at a social occasion. Faced with a beef casserole, elaborately prepared by her host, one vegetarian explained her own panic-stricken reaction: 'I must have forgotten to tell her I was a veggie. I just assume people know. I couldn't really not eat it could I? It was just sat there in front of me.' For others a chance smell of meat cooking evoked not the expected feeling of revulsion but a desire to experience its taste. Bacon was a particular downfall for many vegetarians; one man shrugged apologetically as he said: 'Bacon sandwiches got the better of me.' Steak was also quite commonly mentioned. One vegetarian even had a weakness for raw steak, and on occasion would 'indulge' herself with a dish of steak tartare. Lapses also resulted when people's guard was momentarily down, usually after an evening out which might end up in a burger bar, kebab shop or Indian take-away.

'Lapses' were not necessarily one-off events, rather what defined a lapse was, supposedly, the unpremeditated nature of the meat-eating experience. As one 37-year-old self-defined vegetarian explained of her many momentary lapses:

> About once every three weeks I always have a chicken biriani. I sound like I'm a creature of habit I guess, but at the time it's just something I fancy. . . . Quite often if I've been down the pub and I'm a bit drunk, [I think] 'I could really dig a biriani.'

Vegetarians who defined their meat-eating experience as a 'lapse' were also more likely to have eaten meat outside the home. However, for the majority of vegetarians meat was something prepared by them at home and was a regular part of their diet. Indeed, most people took it for granted that fish, at least, was part of the vegetarian repertoire. For one woman, 'a totally vegetarian meal' included tuna fish, while another said that she was planning to cook fish pie at Christmas, rather than turkey, because: 'The family are all vegetarian.'

Julia Twigg argued that it is 'commonplace' in the process of becoming a vegetarian to give up first red meat, then white meat and finally fish, eating down the 'hierarchy of foods' (1983: 26). However, in South-East London there was little evidence of any patterning in the foods that were given up. For some individuals, red meat, if avoided at all, was the last thing to be renounced rather than the first and there was little sense of having *arrived* at vegetarianism. In those cases in which people described themselves as 'ex-vegetarian' there was also no obvious progression in eating back up the hierarchy. In the same way that some self-defined vegetarians ate the full complement of meats, conversely there were 'meat-eaters' who ate less meat than their vegetarian counterparts. Indeed, many 'meat-eating' participants said they were deliberately reducing their consumption of red meat.

Vegetarianism then, is not a food practice that is rigorously defined, but is a fluid and permeable category embracing a wide range of food practices. It is also an identity that one can dip in and out of. As one woman said: 'I'm often vegetarian apart from the fact that I buy chicken now. . . . I do like chicken curries.'

BEING A 'TRUE VEGETARIAN'

Both vegetarians and meat-eaters were aware of the problems of trying to define vegetarianism. While some individuals had no qualms about calling themselves 'vegetarian', others were more hesitant. Several vegetarians talked of 'true' vegetarianism or 'proper' vegetarianism not just in terms of food consumption, but in the avoidance of all animal products, such as leather, and cosmetics that might have been tested on animals. One woman, a vegetarian for eight years, said 'Sometimes I don't think of myself as a vegetarian at all. Even though I don't eat meat or fish, I do eat dairy produce and I do wear leather shoes so sometimes I don't think I'm a vegetarian.'

However, while some vegetarians in South-East London felt momentary twinges of self-doubt, they accepted their situation with equanimity and expanded their definition of vegetarianism to accommodate aspects of their own diet and lives. The vegetarians were also very accepting of other vegetarians' eating habits. While some might talk in terms of 'proper' vegetarianism, this was as a commentary on their own situation rather than a moral statement about someone else's vegetarian credentials. No sense of elitism existed in which people were seen as better vegetarians the more they avoided animal products. Indeed, in most cases, they were also non-judgemental about the diet of the 'meat-eaters' and did not attempt to proselytise. As a (fish-eating) vegan said: 'I don't think a vegan diet is better than a vegetarian one and if people like eating meat that's fine. Our diet is just better for us, that's all.'

Non-vegetarians, however, were not so lenient. They were more likely to see vegetarian meat-eating as hypocritical and worthy of derision and they enjoyed drawing attention to what they saw as the contradictory behaviour of vegetarians. As one 26-year-old woman said cuttingly: 'My flat-mate calls himself a vegetarian but I don't know how. He eats fish and he's got a bloody fish tank!'

MEAT-EATING AS A CULTURAL TRADITION

Non-vegetarians often felt an imperative to justify their continued consumption of meat. There were several ways in which this was achieved. The first was to minimise the significance of a dietary change. Meat-eating, as such, was frequently couched as a mere 'habit', something of no great importance that, idleness aside, could be given up with ease. 'I've been inclined to want to become a vegetarian', said one 34-year-old secretary, 'but it's just mainly force of habit that I haven't.' Another commented: 'I enjoy meat, I like meat and I wouldn't want to be vegetarian but I could be, I think, without any great difficulty . . . without it being a big problem.'

Others complained that, while attracted to vegetarianism, pressures of work and family life meant they had no time or energy to make the necessary dietary changes. One reluctant meat-eater admitted: 'I have found vegetarian food very long-winded to prepare.' Pressures of time were also used by this woman to excuse her non-vegetarianism: 'Meat is easier to cook. A roast dinner is quick and doesn't take a lot of effort, but nice, tasty vegetarian food takes a while and needs good ingredients.'

For others, this meat-eating 'habit' took on the mantle of an important cultural tradition. Meat was what made a meal and a 'proper meal' always contained it. While much has been written within the social sciences on the cultural importance of the proper meal (Douglas and Nicod 1974, Douglas 1975, Murcott 1982, Charles and Kerr 1988) and in response to the changing nature of food consumption (Fischler 1980, Mintz 1984), the proper meal ideal still had resonance for many people in South-East London. Put simply by a 28-year-old nursery nurse:

> I just don't feel like I'm eating a proper meal if I don't have meat with it. I think it's your upbringing . . . a roast dinner, Shepherd's Pie . . . liver and bacon, as much potatoes and vegetables as you want. Pork chops . . . just all the things you associate with being at home. It's how I see my home: a proper meal.

Such was the cultural importance of meat that some people were genuinely baffled about what vegetarians ate. Some, like this 34-year-old man, while vaguely mumbling about 'rabbit food', concluded: 'I just don't know what I'd eat if I was vegetarian. Everything revolves around the meat, not vice versa.' Indeed, in parodying vegetarianism, others envisaged 'little bowls of boiled lentils or boiled carrots'. Meat-less diets were seen as eminently unsatisfying, both on an emotional and physical level, and some people said they still felt hungry unless they had eaten meat. While vegetarians argued that their diet provided an opportunity for culinary experimentation, they also recognised the significance of meat-based meals. One 29-year-old man said:

> I spend a lot of time trying to adapt vegetarian meals towards that meat and two vegetable ideal. I cook a lot of vegetable pies and thick broths because a lot of vegetarians I know find it comforting to have this old home cooking style food. They get bored with too many bits of fiddly food, which vegetarian food can often be, can't it?

MEAT-EATING AND HEALTH

Meat-eaters also justified their continued consumption of meat on the grounds of health. While current healthy eating guidelines stress a reduction in the consumption of red meat, this did not always correspond with popular opinion about the naturalness of a meat-based diet. One woman in her 40s pointed to our species-given physiology and digestive processes as evidence for the pre-disposition to eat meat: 'By morals and ethics I think I'd like to be vegetarian but I do actually feel that I've got omnivorous teeth and I'm designed as an omnivore.' Others even talked of an innate blood lust. A 20-year-old woman said that: 'You need something with blood, it's important somehow, not just vegs and beans.'

Meat was also considered the primary source of protein and 'trace elements', neither of which could be guaranteed with a vegetarian diet. Consequently, as this man said, danger lay in meatlessness:

> My mother always thought that vegetarianism would kill me and that I would die and that there was no chance I would survive not eating meat. . . . And she always used to buy a little packet of ham just in case.

Ex-vegetarians also saw meat as essential for health. In explaining their return to eating meat, they described craving for meat as a physiological 'need': 'I did try being a vegetarian for a while but I got real cravings for meat lasagne. I don't know if I was missing out on a vitamin or something.' In this context many vegetarian women also saw a craving for meat during pregnancy as a bodily warning sign and would frequently resume eating meat until their baby was born. The fundamental importance of meat was, for many participants, unarguable: 'Meat is mega mega important, there's no two ways about it.'

The unhealthiness of a meat-less diet was also indicated by the physical appearance of vegetarians. They were described as 'pale-looking' individuals who lacked 'any stamina'. During one interview a participant asked my colleague, 'Are you a veggie? I bet you are.' When she acknowledged that yes, she was a vegetarian, he said triumphantly: 'I thought you were . . . you look slightly peaky!'

MARGINALISING VEGETARIANISM: TEENAGE REBELS, CRANKS AND FADDISTS

In defending meat-eating, vegetarianism was frequently marginalised. Lacking any real significance, the move to a vegetarian diet was portrayed particularly by ex-vegetarians as no more than a teenage phase. It was equated with a period of youthful rebellion and was seen as an explicit act of distancing from family life.

Indeed, many parents also talked of their children, 'going through that vegetarian phase'. Vegetarianism thus became a battle of wills between parents and children, as the latter attempted to disrupt established patterns of eating. One woman explained:

> When I became vegetarian my mum said, 'Well if you're gonna be vegetarian then you can cook all your own food.' So I used to make stuff, mountains of it, and I'd have to eat it all week. ... They kept trying to give me meat thinking I would break.

Just as it was common for teenage vegetarians to cook their own food, in many cases they also ate alone. One woman, who became a vegetarian when she was 15 years old, said she did so simply 'to get out of Sunday lunch': the only time when her whole family were guaranteed to be together.

Vegetarianism was also part of the process of political awakening. One teenage vegan, for example, said: 'It was part of a whole thing for me. ... I was marching in London every bloody weekend about something.' In retrospect this dietary change was seen as merely one facet of a youthful and naive idealism: 'I became vegetarian', a 29-year-old explained, 'because I was a lefty, green, ecological sort of half precocious, horrible 16-year-old.'

In adults, however, vegetarianism was seen in a more insidious light, as the practice of cranks and faddists. One man, himself a vegan for the last fifteen years, was well aware of this view. He said:

> Vegan's got a kind of nanu-nanu sound about it. It sounds like you come from a different planet. So I tend to say 'I'm a vegetarian.' Even this isn't always good enough. I come from a working-class Irish meat-and-two-veg family who thinks that vegetarians are a couple of sponge fingers short of a trifle and vegans are some sort of pagan subversives.

As such, vegetarianism can be portrayed as the behaviour of dangerous outsiders. Indeed, throughout the research it became clear that people in general had an antipathy towards what they saw as dietary extremism and hence vegetarianism was seen as an apposite example of 'taking things too far'. It was associated with 'political correctness' and moral earnestness. Vegetarians both lacked a 'sense of humour' and were 'anti-social and withdrawn'. In responding to the question of whether he knew any vegetarians, a 70-year-old man retorted: 'Yes, and I think to myself, "Why don't you have a good lump of meat mate?" They sound to me like a bunch of freaks.' Vegetarianism went against what eating was really all about: enjoyment.

BECOMING A VEGETARIAN

It is surprising that vegetarianism is so marginalised when the majority of vegetarians in this study eat meat, still more when both consumer groups hold broadly similar views on environmental issues such as animal rights and factory farming.

People became vegetarian for a number of different reasons. Some were simply revolted by the taste, texture and appearance of meat which reminded them of its animal origins. Adams argues that to enable the consumer to participate in their consumption, animals become 'absent referents', made invisible through a language which re-names their dead bodies (1990: 40). This process of re-naming, in which pigs become pork and cows become beef, serves to obscure the connection between flesh and food and renders an animal edible.

While Adams's argument fails to account for the vast numbers of animals that are not re-named in this way, for vegetarians in South-East London, the occasion on which the animal origin of meat was acknowledged frequently did mark the point of 'conversion'. For one vegetarian this took the form of a direct correlation between her own body and the flesh of an animal. She said:

> Sometimes you see something in the meat and it would really remind you that it had been another animal. . . . Like your own skin, you know, if you've just got goose pimples and you think, 'Christ, that looks just like chicken skin.'

Squeamish about eating meat since a small child, one 55-year-old woman also said: 'I began to connect that it was flesh, I felt it was like eating your own body.'

However, meat-eaters were not averse to making connections between meat and animals and frequently this also provided the impetus for avoiding certain types of meat. Meat avoided for this reason was usually red meat, the product of larger animals, whose sinews, muscles and bones were more visible. A 40-year-old, who had reduced her consumption of red meat, said: 'Red meat tends to come in big chunks, really, which I don't like very much. Just the, I don't know, the quantity of it. A bit too animal, too obviously animal.' Revulsion at the animality of meat is also reflected, at least in part, in the declining sales of joints of meat in favour of processed meats and meat products. In retailing, the increasing domination of supermarkets at the expense of the traditional High Street butcher's shops, replete with sawdust-covered floors and blood-stained aprons, could also be seen as part of this trend (see Henson 1992).

FACTORY FARMING: 'GOING AGAINST NATURE'

Regardless of their own dietary preference, people wanted to see an improvement in the way animals were reared, transported and slaughtered, calling broadly for a more humane system. For many people in South-East London a confrontation with the realities of factory farming, usually through a television documentary, produced a sense of shock and disgust. Many vegetarians placed the origin of their conversion on such programmes. As one man explained: 'It was that programme on animals and slaughtering. Channel 4 showed it and I couldn't take my eyes off it. The cruelty and everything else. . . . I couldn't take it anymore. I ended up going to the freezer and taking everything out and throwing it away.'

Factory farming was seen simply as unnecessarily cruel and many individuals empathised with the plight of animals caught up in it. As this meat-eating pensioner said:

I can't bear all this business. Seeing all these animals going on to the ships to be transported abroad and they're all huddled together. Just imagine it. They shouldn't be doing that. They should be fed and watered and have regular stops. I wouldn't want to be herded in with a lot of other human beings and not be able to move for several hours. Not being able to move my arms and my legs. Why should we treat animals less well than we treat ourselves?

Such concerns are often used by animal welfare and vegetarian campaigning groups. Publicity materials often gruesomely depict animals' pain and distress, arousing feelings of empathy expressed by this pensioner. In a leaflet entitled 'Why You Should Join the Vegetarian Society' factory farming is emotively described as 'the mass production of misery' (no date: 2). We are told animals:

'spend their brief miserable lives trapped in hideous, artificial conditions, unable to see daylight or to breathe fresh air'. In a 'frenzy of killing brought about by human greed for meat', animals spend their last moments 'in indescribable pain'.

Some vegetarians however were critical of the anthropomorphic sentimentalisation inherent in literature of this kind and were annoyed at the way in which a sympathy for 'fluffy animals with big eyes and wet noses' could effectively distract attention from the real question of the rights of sentient creatures. One vegetarian said somewhat harshly:

> I hate animals. I have no love of animals at all. I don't like them, I don't value their company and certainly don't want them as pets. But I have a respect for the living. I hate cruelty and believe in freedom. I don't think we should give animals the vote but they have a right to a pain-free natural existence.

Yet while a small minority of self-declared 'unashamed carnivores' liked eating meat and shrugged their shoulders in dismissal at suggestions of animal suffering, this was not typical of all meat-eaters. While some participants supported factory farming on the basis that it was the only viable means to provide food for a mass market, even these advocates suggested that some factory-farming practices 'had gone too far'. Common complaints were centred on the use of hormones to fatten animals and on advances in genetic engineering that apparently exceeded the bounds of 'nature'. A 23-year-old student commented that she had stopped eating lamb: 'Because of a newspaper report about hormone treatments making lambs so big that their legs had to be sawn off so that they could be born. I cannot eat lamb after that.'

However, the majority of people were not deterred from eating meat by qualms about killing animals but simply called for a return to the farming practices of 'the past'. Like this meat-eating pensioner, they looked in wistful nostalgia at how things used to be, with 'young chick-a-doodles all running round and the farmer's wife wearing an apron again, like we did during the war'. Rather than being unconcerned with animal welfare issues, people eating meat often did so only when this meat came from free-range or organically reared animals. However, perhaps conscious that this preference might be read as extreme, concerns about 'unnatural' farming practices found expression on a more personal level and were re-written as concerns about the relative taste or safety of such meat for human consumption. Indeed, salmonella in eggs and BSE-infected cattle offered trump cards to be pulled out when disputing the morality of factory farming.

ENVIRONMENTALISM AND MEAT-EATING

In contemporary analyses of vegetarianism, then, eating meat has been seen principally as a symbol of a wider cultural belief in the supremacy of humans over nature. As Fiddes, among others, has argued we have been brought up in a culture that sees environmental conquest as a 'laudable goal' and eating meat as the primary means through which this goal is expressed (1991: 228). Here, meat is given essentially one meaning, as a symbol of the cultural domination of nature.

In a recent history of vegetarianism, looking to the future with undisguised pessimism, Spencer asks whether people 'will ever be able to give up that symbol of human domination over their planet, the slaughtered animal and its carcase meat?' (1994: 343). The symbolism intrinsic to meat, when bound with the sensual, even atavistic pleasure experienced while eating a 'burnt corpse', makes him wary of underestimating the power of the dominant meat-eating culture. Vegetarianism, however, becomes an act of salvation:

> If we want to save ourselves, our children and their future, and this planet that we live on, we must alter our diet radically and rethink our concepts of the living world and the respect and consideration that is ultimately due to it.
>
> (Spencer 1994: 346)

For him, hope lies in the fact that eating meat is also *'habitual'*. As a consequence, abstaining from meat becomes a real possibility (Spencer 1994: 346). Indeed, one teacher in South-East London speculated on the continued growth of vegetarianism and the likely changes this would have on society. Noticing that many of his students were vegetarian he said: 'I have a prediction that in about a hundred years eating meat will be seen as something you don't mention, something obscene. It might not be outlawed, but you'd have to go to special restaurants to eat it.'

In the West, vegetarianism has historically been ridiculed and marginalised. The portrayal of vegetarianism as the diet of 'cranks', 'faddists' or other extremist groups has been read by social scientists as an attempt by the 'dominant culture', to minimise the significance of the social critique inherent in meat abstention: removing meat from the diet challenges the fundamental principles on which society is grounded. Vegetarianism, then, reconceptualises our place in nature and, while meat-eating represents an androcentric attitude, vegetarianism is quintessentially biocentric.

Yet however the future is visualised – as a vegetarian Eden or as a carnivorous Hades – there are fundamental problems in this dualistic premise. As Morris argues in his work on meat-eating in Malawi, there is a 'lamentable tendency' within the social sciences to describe whole cultures in terms of a single motif or paradigm (1994: 22). While dietary choices reflect and reinforce identity, the complexity of this process is hidden when identity becomes simply an issue of the presence or absence of one food item; even more so when this food item, meat, is ascribed only one meaning. Cohen has written on the polysemic nature of symbols that, 'the "*common*ality" which is found in community need not be a uniformity. It does not clone behaviour or ideas. It is a commonality of *forms* (ways of behaving) whose content (meanings) may vary considerably among its members' (Cohen 1989: 20 quoted in James 1993: 207). Following Cohen, then, the position of meat as *the symbol* of an Enlightenment ethic can rightly be called into question.

In South-East London, as I have shown, 'meat-eating' and 'vegetarianism' were expressed and interpreted in numerous ways. This was also true for one locally based environmental group, for whom meat-eating became a tangible expression of a one-ness with nature. This group based their lives on the principles of 'Permaculture'.

The term 'permaculture' was first coined during the late 1970s by two Australian environmental activists, Bill Mollison and David Holmgren (Clunies-Ross and Hildyard 1992, Whitefield 1993: 4). Like many environmental philosophies, at the root of permaculture is a disenchantment with 'the excesses' of modern industrial society and a belief in an impending ecological crisis. As it plunders and pollutes the natural world, humankind is seen as spiralling inevitably towards its own self destruction (Dobson 1992).

Permaculture, however, advocates a sustainable use of the earth's resources:

Permaculture, *perma*nent agri*culture* or *perma*nent *culture*, is the conscious design of a sustainable future based on co-operating with Nature and caring for the Earth and its people. Permaculture ... creates ways of providing for our needs, including food, shelter and financial and social structures.

(South-East London Permaculture 1994)

In permaculture the proselyte finds a philosophy for both the environment and for the self. As one member said, 'I was always dissatisfied with systems we were being offered and I wanted to find an alternative and a practical way of sorting out the environment whilst engaging myself in the process.' What was thought distinctive about permaculture was its emphasis on taking positive and practical steps towards change. Its supporters were critical of armchair-environmentalists who 'talk green and do nothing'. For the South-East London group, 'living a permaculture lifestyle' encapsulated a belief in the ethics of 'earth care, people care and fair shares', but importantly these took practical expression in growing their own organic food, setting up a local wholefood cooperative and working as far as possible within an exchange economy. Many members were also self-employed as permaculture designers (gardeners) and tutors, while others made their own clothes and jewellery from recycled materials.

However, while the majority of members were vegetarian, the group did not advocate vegetarianism as part of a core ideology. They avoided meat because factory farming, like much else in contemporary society, was not a sustainable enterprise. A precondition of resuming a meat-based diet was the certainty not only that animals were reared with reverence and respect, but that the techniques of animal husbandry were environmentally non-destructive. The only way in which this could be guaranteed was to raise one's own animals. Indeed the objective of the majority of the permaculturists was to leave London and set up their own smallholding. As one woman explained: 'I know a lot of people who say when they get on their land they would have chickens and they would eat the eggs and they would eat the meat of whatever livestock they've got.'

Consequently, for members of this environmental group, a meat-less diet did not bring them closer to nature, but was a tangible representation of their alienation from it. Taking responsibility for rearing and slaughtering animals was not barbaric, rather the reverse. It was a means through which the subjectivity of animals was respected and, contrary to Adams's assertion, reversed the process through which they become absent referents. As this permaculturist said:

> I'm not a vegetarian because I'm squeamish about killing animals. . . . What I don't like in this country is the way that animals are herded down long slippery slopes to the whirling blades at the bottom . . . and they're terrified. The [permaculture] farmers will spend a lot of time calming an animal down . . . and they respect it. When I gave up meat I said that I wouldn't eat [it] again till I'd killed something because I didn't like the fact that someone was doing my killing for me. I was just eating a product and that product was something that was once alive and walking around and, you know, having cow feelings.

Eating meat, then, can be a positive way in which to express one's environmental credentials and reflects, not an act of distancing from or domination of animals, but an identification with them. Here, the evidence effectively challenges the trend towards a monosemic reading of meat.

Research in South-East London suggests that vegetarianism does not necessarily involve abstaining from meat and eating meat does not place vegetarians in a precarious moral position, at least in their own eyes. Meat was consumed both as a momentary 'lapse' and also as a regular part of the diet. While meat-eaters were less forgiving of such vegetarian 'indiscretions', the latter readily expanded their own definition of vegetarianism to incorporate the consumption of meat. Indeed, for most participants meat was seen as a central component of a proper meal and was endowed with beneficial properties, both physical and cultural. In comparison to a 'hearty' meat-based meal, vegetarian food was seldom perceived as central to 'family' or 'home'. While food choice is a fundamental component of individual and cultural identity, questions of identity cannot be reduced to the presence or absence of meat in the diet. What is clear is there are no set rules for being a vegetarian, rather individuals define and enact this identity each in their own way.

ACKNOWLEDGEMENTS

The 'Concepts of Healthy Eating' (Lewisham) project was funded by the Economic and Social Research Council as part of its

Research Programme 'The Nation's Diet: The Social Science of Food Choice'. The project was directed by Professor Pat Caplan. Research associates were myself and Anne Keane.

I am grateful to Professor Pat Caplan and Anne Keane for their guidance and comments on various drafts of this paper and to Steve Brace for his unfailing support and encouragement. Most importantly I would like to thank those people who participated in the research and took time to share their experiences.

REFERENCES

Adams, C. (1990) *The Sexual Politics of Meat. A Feminist-Vegetarian Critical Theory*, New York: The Continuum Publishing Company.

Atkinson, P. (1980) 'The symbolic significance of health foods', in M. Turner (ed.) *Nutrition and Lifestyles*, London: Applied Science Publishers.

—— (1983) 'Eating virtue', in A. Murcott (ed.) *The Sociology of Food and Eating: Essays on the Sociological Significance of Food*, Aldershot, Hants: Gower Publishing Company Ltd.

Beardsworth, A. and Keil, T. (1992) 'The vegetarian option: varieties, conversions, motives and careers', *Sociological Review* 40, 2: 253–93.

Caplan, P., Keane, A., Willetts, A. and Williams, J. (1997 forthcoming) 'Concepts of healthy eating: approaches from an anthropological perspective', in A. Murcott (ed.) *Food Choice: Modern Social Science Definitions and Discoveries*, London: Longman.

Charles, N. and Kerr, M. (1988) *Women, Food and Families*, Manchester: Manchester University Press.

Clunies-Ross, T. and Hildyard, N. (1992) *The Politics of Industrial Agriculture*, London: Earthscan Publications.

Cohen, A. (1989) *The Symbolic Construction of Community*, London: Routledge.

Cox, P. (1994) *The New Why You Don't Need Meat*, London: Bloomsbury.

Dobson, A. (1992) *Green Political Thought: An Introduction*, London: Routledge.

Douglas, M. (1975) 'Deciphering a meal', in M. Douglas (ed.) *Implicit Meanings: Essays on Anthropology*, London: Routledge and Kegan Paul.

Douglas, M. and Nicod, M. (1974) 'Taking the biscuit: the structure of British meals', *New Society* 30, 637: 744–7.

Dubisch, J. (1985) 'You are what you eat: religious aspects of the health food movement', in A. Lehmann and J. Myers (eds) *Magic, Witchcraft and Religion: An Anthropological Study of the Supernatural*, California: Mayfield Publishing Company.

Fiddes, N. (1992) *Meat: A Natural Symbol*, London: Routledge.

Fischler, C. (1980) 'Food habits, social change and the nature/culture dilemma', *Social Science Information* 19, 6: 937–53.

Henson, S. (1992) 'From High Street to hypermarket: food retailing in the 1990s', in National Consumer Council (ed.) *Your Food: Whose Choice?* London: HMSO.

Hyde, S., Balloch S. and Ainley, P. (1989) 'A social atlas of poverty in Lewisham', Working Paper (mimeo), London: Centre for Inner City Studies, Goldsmiths' College.

James, A. (1993) 'Eating green(s): discourses of organic food', in K. Milton (ed.) *Environmentalism: The View from Anthropology*, London: Routledge.

Keane, A. and Willetts, A. (1996) 'Concepts of healthy eating: an anthropological investigation in South-East London', Working Paper (mimeo), London: Goldsmiths' College.

Mintz, S. (1984) 'Meals without grace', *Boston Review*, December: 6–7.

Morris, B. (1994) 'Animals as meat and meat as food: reflections on meat-eating in southern Malawi', *Food and Foodways* 6, 1: 19–41.

Murcott, A. (1982) 'On the social significance of the "cooked dinner" in South Wales', *Social Science Information* 21: 672–92.

The Realeat Survey (1984–1995), Conducted by Social Surveys (Gallup) Ltd for The Realeat Company Ltd, London: The Haldane Foods Group.

South-East London Permaculture Group (SELP) (1994) Publicity Flyer: No Title.

Spencer, C. (1994) *The Heretic's Feast: A History of Vegetarianism*, London: Fourth Estate Limited.

Twigg, J. (1979) 'Food for thought: purity and vegetarianism', *Religion* 9: 13–35.

—— (1983) 'Vegetarianism and the meanings of meat', in A. Murcott (ed.) *The Sociology of Food and Eating: Essays on the Sociological Significance of Food*, Aldershot, Hants: Gower Publishing Company Ltd.

The Vegetarian Society (no date) 'Why you should join the Vegetarian Society', Altrincham, Cheshire.

Whitefield, P. (1993) *Permaculture in a Nutshell*, Hampshire: Permanent Publications.

Chapter 7

Urban pleasure?

On the meaning of eating out in a northern city

Lydia Martens and Alan Warde

DINING OUT

> Public dining is an integral aspect of urban living and its relative invisibility as a research topic reflects the extent to which food and eating is a taken-for-granted aspect of everyday life.
>
> (Wood 1992: 5)

The habit of eating out for pleasure has spread to a large proportion of the population. Most people eat out sometimes, many do very often. Thus household expenditure on eating out has risen in the recent past. Eating out absorbed about 10 per cent of household food expenditure in 1960, but 21 per cent by 1993. A recent report (Payne and Payne, 1993) estimated that in 1992 the eating out market was worth £16.6 billion. There are many different ways in which prepared foods are obtained in contemporary Britain. People buy take-away meals and snacks, eat in works canteens, visit family and friends, and buy meals from establishments on whose premises they are eaten. This chapter is concerned with only the last category – with the occasions and sites for eating away from home, where a meal is purchased to be eaten on the premises, in cafes or restaurants.

One of the distinctive features of eating out in a commercial setting is that one does something quintessentially familial – sitting down, for some considerable period of time, at table, to eat – but in the visible presence of strangers. Most commentators have probably interpreted this largely twentieth-century development as a positive one. It has been considered part of a democratic process whereby an activity that was once a luxury restricted to elites has come within reach of the whole population. The value of the place of public refreshment as a site for social participation has often been applauded. The cafe, in particular, has been considered an emblem of democratic political participation, a place where people could discuss political issues and express an opinion about them: Sennett (1976), for instance, saw the eighteenth-century coffee house as a very important training ground for political debate which provided the basis of a public sphere for democratic determination of political issues. Similarly, frequenting public houses has been seen as an important aspect of community solidarity, albeit almost exclusively among men, with a significant role in the mobilisation of political opposition throughout the last 200 years. These were, we should note, places where conversation among strangers was not discouraged.

The presence of strangers in public space might also be welcomed even if it involved a less active participation, for the restaurant provides a location in which the harmonious management of social relations in a public place indicates a degree of mutual tolerance between a wide variety of customers. Sociologists would tend to register this as a counter-tendency to the process of privatisation. Most commentators have thus welcomed the expansion of eating out, so that it may seem perverse of Finkelstein (1989: 5) to claim that 'the practice of dining out is . . . a rich source of incivility'.

Finkelstein's is one of very few books about eating out. However, although she devotes the first half of the book to describing the history of the restaurant, the behaviours involved in eating out, and different types of venue, the purpose of her observations is to apply critical reason to modern culture. *Dining Out* is less an account of eating out, more a critique of the superficiality and lack of self-reflection characteristic of individuals in modern societies with respect to the origins of their desires and reasons for their conduct. Her central thesis is that restaurants are organised in such a way that dining out does not require the 'engagement' of customers in the creation of their own environment of sociality. Thus the decor, service and atmosphere are designed in such a way as to relieve us of the 'responsibility to shape sociality', and this 'weakens our participation in the social arena' (1989: 5). Dining out encourages us to imitate the behaviour of other people in the restaurant, without there being any need 'for thought or self-scrutiny', thus constituting a 'constraint on our moral development' (1989: 5). We are made lazy, because interaction is controlled and we use the ambience of the place to perform a necessary transformation of emotion in ourselves and others, when it should be done instead in an open and engaged way. Thus, elaborating on Elias, she defines civility:

> civilised conduct (i)s that which occurs in exchanges between individuals who are equally self-conscious and attentive to one another, who avoid power differentials and who do not mediate their exchanges through signatory examples of status and prestige.
>
> (1989: 8)

This is to distance herself from common-sense understandings of civilised conduct, which are associated with polite, unemotional and predictable exchanges between people. Indeed, her strongest objections are against unthinking obedience to conventions, a practice easily reproduced by mannered behaviour. Instead she recommends critical self-reflection on personal conduct as a means to weigh the pursuit of private pleasures against moral behaviour oriented to the public good. She considers:

> civility to be a function of the examined life: thus civility cannot be exemplified by an unreflected obedience to habit or custom irrespective of how intrinsically humanitarian the customs are that may emerge from this obedience. Civility is a result of intentional exchange . . . the hallmark of civility is the degree of engagement required of the interactants.
>
> (1989: 9)

So, civility is not the respecting of conventions which facilitate peaceful interaction and exchange of views, but engagement in dialogue without restriction of topic or constraint by authority, rules or orchestration.

For Finkelstein, restaurants fail to offer the circumstances for exchanges of this civilised kind. The regimes of commercial establishments are planned in a way that encourages simulated, rather than genuine, engagement (1989: 52). Conventional behaviour in restaurants amounts to accepting an 'obligation to give a performance in accord with the normative demands of the circumstances' (1989: 53). Such normative demands are conveyed and enforced as part of the operation of a 'diorama', 'that is, a device which heightens and intensifies a manner of perception, the ways in which individuals pursue pleasure and the satisfaction of desire in the practice of eating out' (1989: 27). Subject to the

assorted manipulation of their senses and emotions by establishments providing meals, diners lose both their critical faculties and
their capacities to reflect on their social condition as they accept the
superficial private pleasures associated with restaurants. Since 'the
individual's competent participation in the public [domain] is a sign
of his/her understanding of how social life should be conducted'
(1989: 53), eating out entails that diners, *de facto*, legitimise limited
engagement and limited reflection. Finkelstein thus believes that
expressions of self in public consumption contexts are marked
by superficiality and by lack of opportunity for self-reflection of
the kind that Giddens (1991), for example, maintains is required
by, and is pervasive in, late modernity.

Finkelstein's thesis effectively challenges the authenticity of the
feelings of pleasure reported by people as arising from eating out.
She discredits lay perceptions of the experience:

> Although over the years, from conversations and interviews
> with dozens of regular diners . . . I have collected data on why
> people dine out, and the pleasures they derive, this data has
> always had a limited use. In answer to my question of why dine
> out, the answers were repeatedly that it was fun, a convenience,
> a habit, an entertainment, a pleasure. In answer to any sugges-
> tion to the contrary, with reminders of meals when the food was
> of poor quality or overpriced, when the waiter was intrusive or
> the restaurant too noisy, my respondents most often excused
> these as being rare, circumstantial, and unfortunate. It was not
> admitted that such discomforts may indeed be integral to dining
> out and so should always be expected. . . . a consideration of
> why individuals displayed such limited analytic insight into their
> own conduct suggested, in hindsight, that the process somehow
> thwarted scrutiny.
>
> (1989: 19–20)

Thus she discards reports of experience, believing that diners fail
to see that they are missing opportunities for self-reflection and
self-development.

Finkelstein's account purports to be a case study with general
applicability; dining out is primarily explored in order to illustrate
the more general moral argument. Indeed, the application of the
example of restaurants in the second, theoretical, part of the book
becomes increasingly stretched. Nevertheless, *Dining Out* offers
a brief history of restaurants, a keenly observed typology of

different kinds of eating places, and a plausible analysis of the way that establishments construct ambience to seduce their clients into complicity with the rules of the organisation. Moreover, Finkelstein makes some counter-intuitive but provocative arguments about urban life, social conventions and the pleasures that might be associated with eating out. The rest of this chapter examines some of these positions, particularly with respect to lay perceptions of pleasure among people in the north of England.

EATING OUT IN A NORTHERN CITY: DATA COLLECTION

The data on which this chapter is based was collected through in-depth interviews held with the principal food provider(s) in households diverse in their circumstances. The selection process was similar to that of DeVault (1991: 22), the principal food provider being defined as any 'man or woman who performed a substantial portion of the feeding work of the household'. We conducted thirty interviews, all in Preston and the surrounding area, in the autumn of 1994, each lasting between one and two hours. All interviewees were asked a number of questions relating to the social organisation of eating in the domestic sphere including: work routines, the allocation of tasks, perceptions of change in eating habits over time and food culture. They were then asked about eating out including their understanding of the term, the frequency with which they ate out in various places, details about one recent excursion and a number of attitude questions about eating out. Some questions were asked of all interviewees, but the interviews were of a semi-structured type and topics that seemed likely to increase our understanding of people's food practices were pursued freely. In the next section we examine aspects of the way that our interviewees described and evaluated eating out.

EXPERIENCES OF EATING OUT

Evaluating experiences

Finkelstein argues that due to the power imbalance between restaurant personnel and the diner, the service provider is in a position to 'exploit' the diner in various ways, from overcharging to serving up inferior food. Yet, in their effort to have a pleasurable experience, diners fail to register the negative aspects of the dining experience. Finkelstein's observation that people generally connect eating out with pleasure, and that they are comparatively uncritical, was corroborated in our study. Our respondents generally said they enjoyed eating out. It was relatively difficult to get people to say what they disliked about particular eating out occasions: their first response, as Finkelstein predicted, was often that there was nothing they had disliked about it. Dislikes tend to be, at most, after-thoughts. When asked to recall defective aspects that Finkelstein would consider significant, they may decline to do so, as was the case with Jane.

> *Interviewer*: Do you remember an occasion when you were served bad food?
> *Jane*: No not really. I think we've been quite lucky really. I can't remember.

Yet, even though Jane could not remember negative experiences herself, the mention of 'lucky' by her might suggest that she was aware that others, friends and/or family with whom they discussed these matters, did have negative experiences.

Most people were not unaware of the failings of restaurants but were, rather, very willing to excuse them. For example, Janice reported a 'bar-type' lunch where the food 'was so salty I couldn't eat it', 'some had finished their meal before the others were served', and where they had had to listen to a faulty jukebox for 15 minutes.

> *Interviewer*: Altogether a few hiccups?
> *Janice*: Yeah, yeah, but I mean because of there being a group of us we weren't that concerned really, I mean we quite enjoyed the meal on the whole.
> *Interviewer*: What? Mainly because of your companionship, your friends being there?
> *Janice*: Yeah, yeah.

Reticence in reporting inadequacies was not because people did not register the failure, more that they wished to avoid making the event seem less congenial than it otherwise might have been. Chris, for example, who was interested in food, recounted an occasion where the food was disappointing. Having said that she would not go back, the interviewer asked whether her discontent was discussed at the time. She replied:

Well not at the time because we were, you know, having a nice family outing and so we were talking about various other things. ... But afterwards I said to Norman 'That wasn't really that good was it?' So that was a discussion between him and me afterwards.

Nor was it the case that people were unwilling to complain; some respondents made a point of insisting that when dissatisfied they made their grievances apparent. But this was mostly done discreetly, in a way calculated not to disrupt the order of the restaurant.

Aversion to formal modes of conduct

If Finkelstein's only point was that restaurants are orderly, governed by conventions to which customers mostly accede, then she is surely correct. Many references were made to formal aspects of eating out, indicating an awareness, on the part of respondents, of expected behaviour and treatment in particular establishments. These were, more often than not, accompanied by an assessment of structural aspects of the meal experience, indicating likes and dislikes. Various aspects of the organisation of meals were linked to notions of formality. These included dress, bodily posture, the timing of the eating event and the service and service staff.

In at least one sense, the venue pressurises the client; people think in advance about what it is appropriate to wear. Relaxation is associated with casual dress and formality is identified in terms of the kind of clothing required. But this does not always mean that people will conform to the expectations of the establishment. Rose was discerning about appropriate clothes and discussed at length the relationship between appearance and confidence; for instance, she expressed some admiration for confident people and also sympathy for the view that people should wear what feels comfortable regardless of the occasion. Yet, whilst some respondents were at ease with formal dress codes and rather enjoyed dressing up, others abhorred these demands, and consequently avoided venues and occasions where they felt they had to dress up.

People also registered awareness of rules about bodily demeanour. Putting one's feet up, taking shoes off, and lounging in front of the television, were postures considered unsuitable at a restaurant, but acceptable at the home of friends:

Trisha: Sometimes it's nice to go to a friend's because you don't have to make as much of an effort as if you were going to a restaurant so, and, erm, you can lounge around in front of the tele and, erm, you know, chat and really just relax and sit and chat about *things*.

Pressure of time was a further concern of some respondents who noted that restaurateurs may curtail a meal to suit their own interests. Anne brought this aspect forward as one of her reasons for choosing to eat in bar-type venues rather than in restaurants. Others reflected on the relative informality of eating at the home of friends and family in this respect. Sheila, for instance, thought that eating at the home of friends was a more relaxed affair because you could 'take as long as you like', whilst Andy felt less under the obligation to 'leave at twenty past eleven' when eating at a friend's home.

When pressed, people were most likely to comment adversely on the service, which was variously evaluated in terms of competence, attitudes of staff, speed and potential embarrassment resulting from formality or, conversely, informality. Embarrassment is a term that recurs quite frequently in interviews, indicating awareness of appropriate behaviour by customers and staff. One respondent was aware that occasionally he personally embarrassed people around him. Also socially (rather than technically) inappropriate behaviour by waiters was described on occasion: a husband was given a massage in a restaurant; a waiter failed to direct or lead one woman to her table so that she felt stranded. Children were also seen as a potential source of embarrassment if they 'played up'.

But generally reports suggested limited anxiety about such matters. People seemed fairly comfortable about eating out, perhaps because they go to places that they know and where they know what to expect. Indeed, both the complaints from Janice and Chris noted above were in respect of an unfamiliar venue, and one that had not been their first choice on the relevant occasion.

Preferences and pleasures

In other respects too, and contrary to Finkelstein's view, respondents in our study seemed well able to articulate their reasons for liking some and disliking other restaurants. Many of them thought about commercial eating venues on a continuum from 'better' to 'worse'. Although not the case for everyone, the types of venues considered superior were usually preferred. Some interviewees ate *only* in those places they considered 'better'. Others might prefer to eat in better venues but did not always do so. A third group recognised that venues differed, but regarded each type as relevant for different occasions. The purposes and anticipated pleasures of an excursion are part of the explanation of people's preferences when selecting a place to eat.

Finkelstein attributes variation in experience almost entirely to choice of type of venue. In her view, people go to the place with the ambience appropriate to their purpose, behave in accordance with its associated conventions and hence derive guaranteed, if superficial, satisfaction. We accept that there is some truth to this, but it sorely underestimates the attractions of eating out, which are neither imaginary nor illusory. A better understanding of the remarkable level of satisfaction achieved from eating out would identify different sources of pleasure and thereby throw light on the social significance of the practice.

The pleasures derived from eating out are varied, partly because people have different objectives. Our interviewees identified many kinds of pleasure. Some were what Campbell (1987) would describe as 'traditional'. Traditional hedonism involves the pursuit of pleasures which tend to be instantaneous in their delivery of gratification and which can be regularly repeated without their appeal waning. As Campbell says, 'human beings in all cultures seem to agree on a basic list of activities which are "pleasures" in this sense, such as eating, drinking, sexual intercourse, socializing, singing, dancing and playing games' (1987: 69). When asked about eating out, the food and the immediate company were among the most frequently mentioned reasons for discriminating between places.

Culinary judgements were evident, as with Jane's reflections on one particular aversion:

> I just don't like the Beefeater places. I don't like [places] where you usually do get, well [where the] food's edible, but it's just, you know, things out of a foam packet that are bunged in a pan, you know what I mean? You don't really need a chef to be able to cook, cook those kind of things. Oh and I tell you what [else] I don't like at Beefeater-type places where they give you . . . a

salad which is just a lump of lettuce, a bit of cucumber chopped up on the top and tomato. You know it's not a nice . . . where there's no finesse. I don't like those kind of places.

Chris was also concerned about the quality of the food. Thus she expressed a preference for eating in restaurants rather than in pubs, emphasising that the latter involved eating lower quality food, certainly compared with what she ate at home. But Chris was nevertheless willing to eat in pubs, because of the sociability it generated.

> *Chris*: If we are going out for a Sunday lunch we'll be quite happy to go to our local Boar's Head, where we know a lot of people. The ambience is very nice. The food is not brilliant but it is always good, and it's not, we always say it doesn't taste as good as our own food, do you know what I mean?

Lisa sought even more collective and convivial pleasures, being less concerned with the quality of the food and more with having an entertaining evening out with a large group of friends. As she explained:

> What do I understand by eating out? We eat out as a social gathering. I mean we might not see our friends for six weeks but we'll be going out with them for a meal and that's, we all get together for this meal . . . we always make a point to have a meal, to go out with a gang of us, you know. I mean there can be anything up to eighteen or nineteen of us going out for a meal, and we always try and make a point of having one every six or seven weeks.

Held at places where it was possible to dance after the meal, she gave the impression that food was of limited importance, and that the fun to be had from a night out, occasionally, with a large group of friends was her primary reason for eating out.

Since few eating out events occur without food and companionship, and since these are basic, and therefore reliable, sources of pleasure, then a sure foundation of traditional pleasure will almost always be forthcoming. However, there are a variety of other attractions which usually complement, though sometimes are inconsistent with, the canons of traditional hedonism.

One key element of lay definitions of the term eating out was that it was special, defined in contradistinction to routine and regular behaviour. When discussing whether they would like to eat out more often, a number of interviewees said not, because too frequent repetition of the experience would prevent its remaining special. Thus:

> *Sheila*: Yes, it is more of an event if you don't do it too regularly, yeah. Although sometimes if I do go out to Giacomo's I think, yes, I should come in here once a week for my tea, you know, and treat myself, but, yeah, maybe less frequently would, it makes it more fun if you do it less frequently, yeah.

Pleasure was thus dependent on its being an occasional activity.

An associated concern was with novelty and, particularly, variety. Steve preferred restaurants to pub venues because they offered a more varied menu:

> Pub food tends to be quite similar in most pubs like lasagne or something, or pie and chips, so generally I'd rather go out and eat in restaurants because you can pick a different kind of food to eat.

Others reported liking to try foods that they would not eat at home:

> *Trisha*: I mean I hadn't tried Indian food till about two years ago and when I tried it I thought it was really nice and, you know, there's so many varieties [of food] that you can eat so you should just try different things, even if you don't like them at least you know for [the] future. So we do tend to, especially when we go out, we don't choose the same thing on the menu, you know, every time we go out we tend to, like, go somewhere different and try a different meal and things like that. We get a bit [of] variety.

The search for varied experience, a prominent goal for many people, also extended to seeking out new restaurants and cuisines, something which was most common among those who ate out frequently.

Other social considerations were also relevant. While few people consciously expressed concern about displays of social status, one woman talked about teaching her sons to eat with a view to their future ability to handle formal, public occasions. There were also overtones of social distinction in some of the responses which cited the quality of the food as being one of primary concern. Another woman, while describing the joy of escape from domestic chores, included 'thinking about going out' as an important element of the process, that is anticipating pleasure deriving from the opportunity to eat something different. In Campbell's (1987) terms, this is modern hedonism, because it involves a degree of day-dreaming about anticipated pleasure. However, this was not a very prominent theme in the interviews. Much more frequently mentioned, particularly by women, were the attractions not only of being spared the labour of cooking, but also the luxury of being served by someone else.

The sources of satisfaction from eating out are thus wide-ranging, indicating a mix of traditional and modern urban pleasures. Arguably the traditional pleasures of achieving comfort from food and stimulation from companionship provide a reliable platform from which other, more modern, pleasures may be pursued. Variety, especially, was prized. The range of pleasures anticipated by our respondents confirms the scholarly purpose of exploring lay perceptions of the appeal of eating out. Finkelstein argues that various aspects of the structuring of the meal experience (influenced primarily by the restaurateur) are rarely noticed by the diner and, if noticed, are observed in an uncritical manner without implication for the quality of the experience. However, our interviewees were quite articulate in explaining their preferences for certain eating out establishments. We were able to discern that some were most concerned with the quality (and quantity) of the food, others with a convivial atmosphere, while some sought new and varied experiences, and yet others simply relished being served. These objectives, along with their perceptions of formality, partly determined the choice of venue.

Varieties of meanings

Finkelstein attributes variation in experience almost entirely to choice of type of venue, whose conventions then structure behaviour. This assumes that everyone shares a common understanding of the nature of the place visited. Four of our respondents commented, at some length, about their experiences of eating at the 'Tavern Fayre', a comparatively recently opened establishment situated on the outskirts of the city. It was described as a large pub which catered in different spaces (and times) for different clientele, there being both a bar area and a separate restaurant where children were allowed. Three of our respondents, Jenny, Katrine and Meg, viewed it positively. Jenny and Meg had been there a number of times and had enjoyed those occasions. Jenny's account in particular highlighted the good points: everything was good, the service, the food and the decor. Thus:

> *Jenny*: Yeah it's really good and it's really good food as well. 'Cos I don't know how they cook it because it's, I mean they don't cook it before you get there but ten minutes and your meal's there. It's really clean as well and you get lots. You get really good value for your money. Your plate is absolutely stacked. They don't skimp on anything.
> *Interviewer*: So they make an effort?
> *Jenny*: Yeah.
> *Interviewer*: What is the decor like in there?
> *Jenny*: Very, very plush, very nice. All the windows, it's all swags and tails curtains. It's very, like, open brickwork. You get lots of features inside. And it's very nice, it's really, really nice.

Rose had also visited the same place on a number of occasions but had become less positive as time went on. In general, it should be said, Rose displayed a more critical awareness about public eating. According to her, the first impressions were good, but recurrent visits would make its limitations obvious to the discerning customer.

> I mean Tavern Fayre as I mentioned before is just up the road. And I think we've been on three maybe four separate occasions, and it is quite cheap, you do get quite a lot. As I say I've been four times now and more or less exhausted the menu and once you get over the fact that you get quite a lot to eat there, I don't think the quality of the food is (*Interviewer*: 'Great?') No, not really, it's quick sort of turnover. It's obviously not freshly cooked because they wouldn't have time to do it. I think it's sort of microwaved or however they heat it up and pretty bland. But the menu I don't think has changed since the place has opened.

Later, when discussing the quality of the food served in eating out places, she talked again about this venue. Rose enjoys eating foods in restaurants which she cannot, or does not, cook at home:

Sometimes it's, um, it tastes a bit mass-produced depending on where you go. I mean the stuff at the Tavern Fayre I could do, reproduce that, stuff like roast beef and Yorkshire pudding and roast potatoes. That's something that we have anyway . . . so I tend to avoid that. But it's not a very extensive menu. I think it's a case of, as I say it's like a glorified pub lunch, which has quite a nice interior and the service isn't too bad. But I wouldn't go really for a special occasion.

Thus it would seem the pleasure derived from an eating out event depends not only on the place itself, but also upon the understandings and interpretations of the participants. Jenny and Rose clearly have different expectations, different criteria of judgement, and are not impressed in the same way by similar food, service or decor. This means that, at the very least, the arrangement of the restaurant by its management does not determine entirely the experience of the customers. The effects of the diorama are limited and various.

REFLECTIONS ON EATING OUT AND INCIVILITY

The principal purpose of *Dining Out* is not to account for eating out, but rather to offer a critique of the superficiality of ordinary conduct if not subjected to eternal self-examination. As such, the value of an empirical critique of the argument as applied to the restaurant is limited. However, given the astuteness and accuracy of many of Finkelstein's observations, it is worth trying to evaluate the causes of the conventional behaviour involved. As Wood (1994) has commented, it is not entirely clear what Finkelstein believes is the root cause of imperfect sociality in restaurants. Is the shallow sociality described as an inevitable effect of meetings in public space, thus implicitly recommending the virtue of private interaction and domestic life? Or is it the consequence of commodification and consumerism, the requirement of the patron who seeks to control and manipulate clients the better to maintain order and increase profits? Or is the incivility inseparable from modern urban culture, in its most general aspects, where all activities open to the scrutiny of strangers exhibit the traits of Simmel's metropolitan mental life? Examination of this ambiguity further clarifies the nature of eating out.

Eating out as a differentiated experience

We have some sympathy with Finkelstein's search for critical self-reflection on personal conduct, which is a *sine qua non* of radical thought and action. Moreover, the idea of the examined life, and its role in the construction of a coherent sense of self, problematises purely expressive accounts of consumption. By advocating the examined life, and by postulating reasoned moral standpoints with respect to all aspects of mundane conduct, Finkelstein is sailing against the tide of current social theory. Much of her argument works by contrasting the *appearance* of pleasure, derived from the world of commodities and display, and the real foundation of the engaged, social and moral self. Her key point is that the expressive aspects of consumer behaviour are generally to be deplored because they inhibit self-reflection and moral development. If this is the current predicament, it becomes difficult to understand why, when pleasures are fragile and imaginary, people generally continue to consume so relentlessly and with so much apparent commitment. Finkelstein's only recourse is to an explanation in terms of subconscious manipulation.

On the basis of our interview material we dispute Finkelstein's readiness to dismiss people's own accounts of their experiences of eating out. Some of her predictions about responses are well founded: people are indeed inclined to give optimistic interpretations of their excursions, for instance. She is also correct in observing that the conventions of different establishments do constrain the behaviour of customers, otherwise there would be greater opportunity for embarrassment and presumably the restaurant would be a much less orderly environment than it normally is. But whether one should regret the existence of those conventions, or suggest that if only diners were more reflective they would opt for alternative courses of action, is debatable. The argument, like others that seek a remoralisation of behaviour, hovers on the edge of attributing to the lay actor a false consciousness. To attribute false needs or consciousness is permissible only under certain very restricted circumstances: where one can identify people's interests unambiguously, where one can clearly identify the mechanism creating such consciousness, and where one can demonstrate that the mechanism actually has the effects postulated (see Lukes 1974). The devices associated with the diorama are in principle an appropriate mechanism for explaining the emergence of incivility. However, the responses of our inter-viewees give only weak support to the actual achievement of the effects of the diorama; people are not so obviously misled.

The various sources of pleasure reported imply that diners are discerning people, who actively participate in and shape the event, rather than being confused, blinded or de-sensitised by the regime of the establishment in which they find themselves. When asked why they go to places, people give different answers. Some go because of the food. Others go because of the company, because it is an opportunity for sociability and conviviality; for them the food is a matter of comparative indifference. Some go to avoid domestic labour, some just for a change. Some people, rather than being intimidated into polite inauthenticity by their surroundings, do not even notice the decor, or the staff, or the other customers. Different people read the signs and symbols in different ways: they understand the same place differently, a point which has been extensively demonstrated in much recent cultural geography.

Perhaps Finkelstein relays the experience and understanding of one section of the population as if it were universal. She projects onto others, of different ages, class and experience, a cosmopolitan and perhaps 'new petit bourgeois' (in Bourdieu's, 1984, sense) view of the activity of eating out. It seems likely that attitudes to food are class specific. DeVault (1991), for instance, depicts a discourse about food that is particular to middle-class Americans. There it is expected that such people will be able to talk articulately about foods and restaurants, even when they are little interested in the topic, since it is a part of the cultural capital required in some circles (Erickson 1991). The consequent danger is that the articu-late project on to others their own impressions, to the extent that it is not considered worth talking to other people, or believing what they say, or asking about their sources of enjoyment, because this is already deemed to be self-evident.

Private behaviour in public places

One of Finkelstein's contributions is, precisely, to problematise dominant evaluations of public space. At least part of the time she seems to imply that because public interaction is governed by convention it will be inherently unsatisfactory. It is hard to interpret her as saying anything other than that it is better to eat in private, since social interactions in private places are more authentic because less open to intrusion or interference. Apart from suggesting a very pessimistic future for an increasingly urban world, this seems to be out of accord with, or rather to misjudge, the significance of public space.

If Finkelstein's utopia is the private, domestic, introspective episode of self-examination, others hold contrary views, expecting positive social benefits from participation and interaction in public space. However, neither of these alternative aspirations are apparently realised in the restaurant. One observable trait of behaviour in restaurants is that people at different tables rarely engage in conversation with one another. The restaurant is not exactly a public place, rather it is a quasi-public place. The restaurant is a space containing a number of private reservations (tables), from which mutual inspection of the tenants of other reservations is permitted, and where one's own behaviour is restrained by the gaze (and power) of others. So, eating out is not necessarily commendable for its encouragement of public conviviality and coexistence. Rather it is private behaviour in a public place. To that extent, it has limited potential for encouraging a public sphere or civil society. However, it does have some other, if less elevated, functions for customers.

Appadurai (1988), talking of the emergence of a national cuisine in India, notes that:

> eating permits a variety of registers, tied to particular contexts, so that what is done in a restaurant may be different from what is appropriate at home, and each of these might be different in the context of travel, where anonymity can sometimes be assured. . . . The new cuisine permits the growing middle classes of Indian towns and cities to maintain a rich and context-sensitive repertoire of culinary postures. . . .
>
> (1988: 9)

Finkelstein, by contrast, fails to appreciate that the culinary postures associated with eating out might be worthy of celebration. Thus factors which she highlights – the opportunity of seeing others and being seen associated with grazing, eavesdropping on other people's conversations, anonymity, wallowing in acknowledged artificial pleasures, pretending to be whoever you want, partaking of a non-binding ritual – may all be harmless sources of pleasure offered by the protected, quasi-public spaces of the restaurant.

Restaurants offer possibilities and opportunities for a somewhat sanitised version of the urban experience, a dip into the maelstrom of modernity, without being exposed to too much danger. This sanitisation entails some compromise: abiding by the rules of the owner, subjecting oneself sometimes to some irksome conventions in order to ensure the preconditions for the obtaining of pleasure from the mutual gaze. But this may be worthwhile, and indeed may be a source of tolerance in its own right.

While restaurants may fail to live up to the hopes of collective conviviality among strangers, it is doubtful whether other contexts for eating are any more likely to guarantee socially beneficial outcomes. Perhaps Finkelstein ought to conclude it best if people ate alone, for we seriously doubt whether domestic situations are any more conducive to civility than are restaurants. Household meals have rarely been characterised as 'exchanges between individuals who are equally self-conscious and attentive to one another, who avoid power differentials and who do not mediate their exchanges through signatory examples of status and prestige' (Finkelstein 1989: 8). Domestic eating is scarcely less regulated or 'managed' than are meals in restaurants. Indeed, it might be argued that many of the apparently uncomfortable aspects of eating at restaurants themselves have their origins in the constraints associated with private hospitality.

CONCLUSION

Our research suggests a number of qualifications and corrections to Finkelstein's arguments in *Dining Out*. Her attempt to use dining out as a metaphor for the experience of modernity is overstretched, leading her to make a series of unsupportable claims about the practice of eating out. The experience of eating out is neither as homogeneous nor as passive as she implies. Different kinds of people seek different sorts of pleasure when they eat out; the fact that they all seem to obtain pleasure should not be interpreted in terms of their having been duped by restaurateurs deploying surreptitious techniques of control, but in terms of socially grounded expectations concerning the sources of enjoyment. Finkelstein's most fundamental mistake is to underestimate the social variation in the creation and appreciation of pleasures. In general people are discerning, self-conscious, and aware of the various elements of the experience of eating out and thus can talk about them in discriminating fashion. They are capable of identifying the inadequacies of a particular meal out, though they are frequently prepared to overlook, or accommodate, such deficiencies. Eating out might not only be viewed as genuinely pleasurable, but also as a welcome alternative to the privatisation of social life, for the restaurant is a comparatively safe, quasi-public environment in which to enjoy many of the real, if ambivalent, attractions of modern urban experience.

ACKNOWLEDGEMENTS

We gratefully acknowledge support for this research from the Economic and Social Research Council, under the auspices of its Programme, 'The Nation's Diet: The Social Science of Food Choice'. Earlier versions of this chapter were delivered at the British Sociological Association annual conference in Leicester in April 1995 and at the European Sociological Association conference in Budapest in September 1995. We are grateful for the constructive comments of participants.

REFERENCES

Appadurai, A. (1988) 'How to make a national cuisine: cookbooks in contemporary India', *Comparative Studies of Society and History* 13: 3–24.

Bourdieu, P. (1984) *Distinction: A Social Critique of the Judgment of Taste*, London: Routledge and Kegan Paul.

Campbell, C. (1987) *The Romantic Ethic and the Spirit of Modern Consumerism*, Oxford: Blackwell.

DeVault, M. (1991) *Feeding the Family: The Social Organization of Caring as Gendered Work*, Chicago: Chicago University Press.

Erickson, B. (1991) 'What is good taste for?', *Canadian Review of Sociology and Anthropology* 28, 2: 255–78.

Finkelstein, J. (1989) *Dining Out: A Sociology of Modern Manners*, Cambridge: Polity.

Giddens, A. (1991) *Modernity and Self-Identity*, Cambridge: Polity.

Lukes, S. (1974) *Power: A Radical View*, London: Macmillan.

Mennell, S. (1985) *All Manners of Food: Eating and Taste in England and France from the Middle Ages to the Present*, Oxford: Blackwell.

Payne, M. and Payne, B. (1993) *Eating Out in the UK: Market Structure, Consumer Attitudes and Prospects for the 1990s*, Economist Intelligence Unit Special Report No. 2169, London, Economist Intelligence Unit and Business International.

Sennett, R. (1976) *The Fall of Public Man*, Cambridge: Cambridge University Press.

Wood, R. (1992) 'Dining out in the urban context', *British Food Journal* 94, 9: 3–5.

Wood, R. (1994) 'Dining out on sociological neglect', *British Food Journal* 96, 10: 10–14.

Chapter 8

'We never eat like this at home'

Food on holiday

Janice Williams

THE SOCIAL, PSYCHOLOGICAL AND PHYSICAL BODY: HEALTH AS CONTROL AND HEALTH AS RELEASE

> Power would be a fragile thing if its only function were to repress . . . in a negative way. If, on the contrary, power is strong this is because . . . it produces effects at the level of desire.
>
> (Foucault 1978: 59)

In recent decades 'health' has increasingly become a matter not only of government campaigns but of mass and self-conscious preoccupation, so much so that Crawford (1984) states that in secular disenchanted western society it is for some tantamount to salvation; 'health' becomes no less than the measure of personhood. 'The biomedical definition of the self is encoded as a cultural program with health as its personal, medical and political objective' (1984: 62). While he locates the reasons for this ascendancy in a real and proper concern for depredations on the environment and a disillusionment with the possibilities of biomedicine, one of his main arguments is that 'health' has become increasingly seen as a matter for self-control and self-discipline, epitomised, for example, in the campaigns that we should smoke less, eat less red meat and take more exercise. Such a moralistic tenor of 'health as self-control' can be both self-validating and guilt-inducing. As Crawford shows from his interview material, those who judge themselves in such terms also judge others by the same criteria, so that those who do not conform are somehow deemed morally inferior. In western notions of self and personhood, 'health' thereby becomes a means for personal and social evaluation.

Crawford also argues that 'health as self-control' is especially typical of the middle classes, for whom the values of self-creation and self-improvement are so important. For the working classes, on the other hand, the value of labour tends to be an end in itself and the main measure of personhood. Alluding to the work of Weber, Elias, Foucault, Freud and Marcuse on the rise of bourgeois individualism and the kind of modal personality structure required by the Protestant work ethic, Crawford demonstrates how for the middle classes, such an ethic, under the rubric of 'health as self-control', becomes extended to the human body. Indeed, the Protestant world-view also invades the domain of leisure in the form of a constant barrage of keep-fit campaigns. The assumption is that there must of necessity be some congruence between the social body, the psychological body and the physical body. Thus health is no longer something to do with inheritance or luck, but rather an achieved status which must be worked on and striven for. For the middle classes, discipline and self-control are involved, particularly in a conservative political climate where former means of self-validation, such as job security and an assured income, can no longer be taken for granted as a measure of status.

Drawing from Foucault's work (1978), Crawford notes that if culture normally represses sexual expression, it also provides for its desublimation. Every culture organises releases from its normal renunciations or 'moral demand systems', as instanced by festivals, holidays, ecstatic religious experiences, intoxications, war, pogroms, sport and games. While celebrations of release can turn against the social order, typically release is a means by which societal tensions are managed. In contemporary American culture, he argues, release is not only an essential mode of relieving pressure that otherwise might not be contained, but also the indispensable creed of its economic system. Release has been appropriated to the requirements of consumption. In the second half of his article he concentrates on the symbolic modality of the salubrious qualities of 'health as release', logically entailed in the opposite concept of 'health as self-control'. Crawford notes that the interplay between self-control and release, apparent within individuals as well as within society, 'reveals an underlying symbolic and structural order, a logic of "freedom" and constraint which in advanced capitalist societies is inherent in the contradiction between production and consumption'.

It is important to note that in the conception of 'health as release', health is more likely to be understood in psychosomatic rather than purely physical terms and also that 'health as release' and the attempt 'not to worry' can begin to sound like a discipline. In Crawford's interpretation, the advocates of release are not necessarily, therefore, more 'free' than the advocates of 'restraint', and repression is well-nigh pervasive.

Crawford links consumption (and therefore eating) to health, and places both topics within the wider context of a political economy of health. Drawing on Mary Douglas's seminal ideas regarding the physical and social body (1966, 1970), for Crawford the body is culturally constructed and the imposition of cultural categories makes it difficult to know where nature ends and culture begins. Anthropological studies of bodily experience, mediated through the symbolic categories of illness and health and including beliefs surrounding food, attempt to uncover the semantic and social structures through which experience is organised in a culture. Alluding to the work of T. Turner (1980), he notes that beliefs and practices concerning the body are particularly instructive because they are located on the common frontier of society, the social self and the psychological individual. As will be shown, talking about health and eating reveals tacit assumptions about individual and social reality.

Although the questions posed in interviews were by no means identical, such is the resonance of some of my own findings with those of Crawford's research on lay notions of 'health' in American (Chicago) culture that in this article I attempt to indicate the extent to which his interpretation is applicable to the UK in general and to research carried out in South-West Wales in particular.

Of particular relevance to the concerns of this article are his identification and interpretation of the symbolic modalities of 'control' and 'release' as major conceptual vehicles whereby 'health' is given expressive form in American culture. In this article, I consider these concepts in analysing interviews conducted with tourists visiting South-West Wales, and discussing the contrasts between what they eat on holiday, and what they eat at home.

THE RESEARCH LOCATION AND THE INTERVIEWS

The development of tourism as a major economic and social phenomenon in the course of the second part of the twentieth century has reached such proportions that it would be surprising if this did not have an impact on western psychological structure. Leisure is big business, tourism accounting for 4.0 per cent of the GDP of the UK economy in 1995 and 5.2 per cent GDP (£1.6 billion) of the Welsh economy, where it accounts for almost one in ten jobs.[1] In Newport (Pembrokeshire), in South-West Wales, where research for this article was conducted,[2] tourism is second only to agriculture in contributing to the local economy.

Newport is a small seaside town which is often described as the 'Jewel in the Crown' of the Pembrokeshire National Park in Wales. This article is mainly based on 23 interviews with 'tourists' or 'visitors' which took place in 1994 during the height of the main tourist season which falls between the end of July and the second week of September, when the population of the town quadruples with the influx of tourists, day-trippers and the return of second-home owners.[3] During 'the season', as it is known locally, there is a sense of frenetic activity in the town which stands in marked contrast to the comparative quiet of the winter months. My field-work diary for this period is packed with references to numerous events and festivities, many involving food. While one of the dominant themes to emerge from interviews with holiday-makers is that they explicitly come to escape the 'stress' of their daily working lives, it is the turn of local tradespeople, caterers and retailers, working long hours under intense pressure, to experience it instead.

Contacts with tourists/visitors were initiated through enlisting the help of owners/managers of local guest-houses, hotels, restaurants and cafes and by approaching people on the spot. Interviews took place where people were staying, at my own field-work base and cottage, on beaches and caravan sites, in restaurants, cafes, and pubs and at a carnival. This indicates a great strength of the anthropological approach of participant-observation; it is possible to obtain very different data on the theme of food on holidays if the interviewees are actually on holiday at the time, than might otherwise be the case. The length of the interviews varied greatly, with ten interviews lasting an hour or longer, and the remainder being somewhat shorter. The majority are joint interviews, half involving both parents of nuclear families who had come on holiday with their children; in many cases the children joined in or were present at the interviews as well. Other interviews involved extended families, couples, friends, and varying combinations of relatives. The total number of adult tourists/visitors interviewed aged 20 and over was forty-five.

While I approached all interviews with a list of topics to be covered, I also tried to be flexible and followed up cues from informants themselves so as to pursue themes which were important to them. I limited the main topics covered to the role of food on holidays, the differences between eating on holidays and eating at home, healthy eating and, if time permitted, the informant's perspective on good food and healthy food. In addition, wherever possible, I tried to obtain some basic socio-economic background data on informants, along with trying to establish why they had come to the town, length of stay, frequency of visits, type of accommodation and reason for the choice of specific accommodation.

Most tourists interviewed were English, from the South, South-East, Midlands or North of England and in the remaining six interviews the participants were all Welsh from other parts of South Wales. Where possible, interviewees' own definitions of class position were sought, while in terms of occupational status, there was a preponderance of people in white-collar, middle-class jobs, and in only seven or eight of the interviews did the participants have manual, blue-collar jobs. In half of the interviews both partners worked full-time. The ages of the interviewees ranged from people in their 20s and 30s to those who were middle-aged and older.

The majority of these tourists visit the town and area for holidays or weekend breaks during the summertime. Most of them had visited the area regularly for a period of at least five years, and participants in seven of the interviews had done so for anything between sixteen and thirty years. On being asked why they had come on holiday to Newport, many informants referred directly or indirectly either to the beauty of the natural landscape in the area or its peacefulness and quietness and the fact that it is uncommercialised and 'not touristy'. Activities on holiday were wide-ranging, and included going to the beach, wind-surfing, canoeing, fishing, boating, sailing, golf, walking, cycling, pony-trekking, and visiting historic sites, craft places and agricultural shows. The majority of interviewees were accompanied by children and parents felt that it gave them an opportunity of bringing children, as one interviewee put it, 'back to the basics you know – you've got the beach – the natural things'. Another noted that: 'this is much more like *my* childhood . . . and they really enjoy it – it's freedom'. Another mentioned that: 'Time stands still here for us', and many contrasted the pace of life in the area with the pace of life in an urban environment:

> *Stepmother*: . . . the area is unspoiled – it's pretty.
> *Stepdaughter*: Pace of life as well – it's lovely! Come day, go day, God send Sunday, and just carry on slowly doing what you want at your own pace, and don't rush it.

For another family, living in London was 'a rat-race' and visiting the area once every six weeks 'keeps the lid on' and 'keeps us sane'. As I shall elaborate below, some of these tourists therefore explicitly contrasted the pace of their working lives with taking a break or being on holiday.

THE IMPORTANCE OF FOOD ON HOLIDAY

Undoubtedly reflecting the shift in importance from bed and breakfast to self-catering in recent years, approximately two-thirds of these interviewees were staying in self-catering accommodation, while the remainder were staying at hotels, pubs cum hotels, or guest-houses which frequently had attached restaurants. A very small number involved second-home owners and a locally born woman returning for her summer holiday. Half the self-caterers (six interviews) had rented cottages or houses and the other half (seven interviews) were staying in caravans, some of which had very basic cooking facilities while others were extremely well-equipped.

Although no informants gave food as a reason for choosing the town or area, several stated that food is important on holiday and for some, 'good food', along with the welcome they received, constituted a major deciding factor in choosing a particular hotel or guest-house. For the participants in one interview, food on holiday was 'very important' and they had selected their hotel on the grounds that it had 'good food' and a pool for the children:

Wife: Well the food here is exceptionally good. It's all very wholesome food.
Daughter: Presentation.
Wife: There's nothing processed or –
Husband: Nice fresh cooked honest meals.
Wife: . . . [no] convenience or anything about it. You know, it's virtually prepared as you're going to eat it.
Son: And the staff make you feel welcome as well.

The welcome received and the food was also important for another family which had stayed regularly for seven years in the same guest-house which had a restaurant of good reputation. In this interview the wife explained why they really enjoyed eating out on holiday:

> It's a treat to come somewhere where there is really excellent food and it's very relaxing just to have dinner and to know that somebody else is washing up. Yes it is a treat and we might not appreciate it quite so much if we ate out all of the time, so it *is* nice for us.

As with other interviews, there is a significant contrast in pace and time between food in the course of daily working life and food on holidays. This theme of the way in which leading very busy working lives impinged on activities surrounding the purchase, preparation and eating of food at home emerges from a significant number of the interviews reviewed in this chapter.

Some informants perceived catering at home and self-catering on holiday as quite different. One tourist stated:

> One of the reasons I don't mind self-catering . . . I actually like cooking but what I don't like is working full-time and running a house and cooking and then never having time to do it properly – but actually cooking on holiday when all you're doing is going to the beach or for a hike and coming home and cooking a meal – well, I quite like that – and it's nice here because you can get things like crab and salmon.

This quotation suggests an implicit distinction between, on the one hand, cooking 'properly' for recreation and, on the other hand, cooking as a chore without enough time to do a good job of it. The same interviewee, on being asked what kind of things she cooked at home, stated:

Well, the trouble is that my repertoire of recipes is huge but what I actually cook for dinner at night after work – huh [laughs loudly] is fairly standard. We eat quite a lot of pasta of various kinds. . . . I'm often conscious that I don't cook an enormous range except on Saturdays when I might be a bit more adventurous and take a bit more time.

She confirmed that she was quite tired at the end of the day's work, 'so you tend to churn out the same repertoire you know'. One married couple agreed that on holiday they ate less convenience food: 'Because we tend to eat very late and we are both very busy we rely an awful lot on lean cuisine when we're at home . . . [and this could go] straight into the microwave.' Other interviewees also alluded to relying heavily on convenience meals and take-aways at home or to cooking food in batches during holidays and freezing it as strategies for coping during busy working weeks.

In one interview, it is apparent that for the rest of the year, cooking time competes with precious time for recreation for people leading busy working lives.

> *Husband*: Sunday really is a time for relaxation. . . . And I think now we always take advantage of as much as we can on a Sunday. When we eat it develops into a late breakfast – brunch – and then the rest of the day if it's going to be spent recreationally –
> *Wife*: Don't want to spend it cooking.
> *Husband*: No – no way.
> *Question*: No. OK, does that spill over in your holidays? . . . I mean the general idea that it's for recreation and you don't want to be too bothered with cooking in your caravan?
> *Wife*: Yes.
> *Husband*: Yes, very much so, I would have thought so.

Behaviour surrounding food preparation and consumption at weekends is thus similar to that on holiday in some respects, although different families allocate different priorities to food during times of relaxation, whether these be at weekends or on holiday. What is striking about the quotation just cited is the way in which there is a definite hierarchy of values, with recreation being placed high and cooking low on the list. The same theme emerges from another interview with self-caterers, the wife stating:

Wife: We're in a caravan so all the food which we eat generally has to be quick – and we're on holiday – so those two are important factors – we've only got a limited space to cook in and we're on holiday so I don't want to spend a lot of time cooking so it all has to be sort of quick easy cooking – instant . . . holiday food is as less work as possible . . . out of a packet.

'Tins', the husband volunteered.

Making time for recreation can thus be as powerful a factor as the demands of work in determining the choices made by tourists around food, and cooking itself can fall into either category.

There was often a difference in time structure between eating at home and eating on holiday. For one family, because they were staying at a hotel, eating was perceived as far more structured than the pattern at home and therefore to be enjoyed and savoured. By contrast with those mothers who were staying in hotels because it was a holiday for them from cooking and shopping and who therefore found it a 'treat' and 'relaxing' to have someone else do the work, for self-catering mothers with young children holiday times could be stressful, as the woman in the following interview graphically observed:

Question: You said that 1988 was wonderful – what was wonderful and accounted for the switch from self-catering to hotel?

Wife: I mean the stress and the pressure, I mean. I don't know whether you've got a young family but self-catering to me – it's not a holiday. At all. I mean when you've breakfasts to cook and lunches to sort out, packing up lunches. They're coming out, coming home, off the beach or wherever you've been and you've got to start thinking about cooking again. Because at that stage when the children were young we couldn't really even afford to eat out. When we was in the caravan we cooked at night, you know, had a meal. So it wasn't really much of a break. Although it was because I didn't know any different. It's what I'd done as a child, what my parents had done for me and I did exactly the same for my children. So it wasn't a chore until I had a taste of actually going into a hotel and being waited on hand and foot and that is when, you know. Really felt as though I'd had a holiday. It was super, it really was and everybody was so much more relaxed, I mean *it was*.

Those who had opted for self-catering accommodation had frequently done so because they had children and in one case a dog. Hotels were seen as more formal than self-catering, and 'with youngsters', as one man noted, 'you're a bit on your guard – you say don't do this and don't do that.' Children were obviously more at ease in informal settings, a point echoed by another interviewee who noted: 'Teenage boys are more comfortable going somewhere fairly casual.' In some cases the children were very young, and mothers stated that self-catering was easier.

An equally important consideration in opting for self-catering was cost. One working-class mother, for instance, said that eating out on holiday, as well as choosing anything other than self-catering, was ruled out by the cost of feeding her five children. They had all their meals in their caravan. Reflecting the economic crises of the times in which we live, one middle-class professional man stated they had chosen self-catering in a caravan because of the price as well as the flexibility, noting that even in his comparatively well-paid profession, many of the people he knew were doing the same thing in 'adjusting to a different economic climate'. Price and the formality of hotels/guest-houses were also mentioned by another father, while his wife also commented on the cost of eating out on holiday when a group of four was involved. Self-caterers with children who did eat out tended to choose pubs, which were of major importance in catering to their needs during the summer holidays – a fact which could scarcely be ignored by even a casual observer, for their doors would be bursting at the seams and full of family groups.[4]

The contrast between food during holiday time and food during working lives becomes combined with another contrast: eating to re-fuel and eating for pleasure. One woman explained her husband's views: 'Well, as I said, he eats for pleasure – he doesn't always eat to re-fuel and he likes a place that he gets a feedback – atmosphere. . . . He'll sit at a table for five hours.' Her remarks were made in the context of a discussion in which it became clear that for her husband enjoyment of good food was not the only requirement of having a good night out. It had to be, as he himself put it, 'Nicely presented – in nice surroundings that I – I could go to a lot of places and eat, but not where I would want to sit and hold a conversation and hold a chat, and be nicely served.' The images presented are not simply those of enjoyment, but also of sociability.

Some visitors, however, did classify their eating as re-fuelling:

Question: . . . the main reason you've come here isn't for the food – the main reason is the walking?
Father: Yes.
Mother: Yes, though we thought the food might be important [laughing] – but it's become less important.
Son: Well, because we're walking a lot we just seem to like *lots* of food – we don't really mind what we're eating somehow.
Mother: In the evening – yeah – in the evening we need it, don't we – we all feel hungry. Breakfast we could do without. [laughing]
Question: That's interesting what you've [Son] just said because you're so hungry that you eat anything and other times when you're not so hungry?
Son: Yeah at home we wouldn't –
Mother: We'd be more discerning, wouldn't we, normally –
Son: There'd be more cooking.

This family was doing a great deal of exercise whilst on holiday, a pattern that was uncharacteristic of their lives at home. In another nuclear family with teenage children, the mother stated that on holiday they were 'sailors and windsurfers', stressing that the food they ate was '*masses* and not expensive' since everyone was using up a lot of energy and was constantly hungry. In both these interviews, therefore, there is a correlation made by the participants between exercise, hunger and quantity. There is an explicit association between hunger and lack of discrimination in the quality as opposed to the quantity of food.

From the data in this and other interviews, it is possible to make the further inference that when one is hungry there is a weakness in the normal boundaries between acceptable and unacceptable food, particularly when one is outside one's normal surroundings as on holiday:

Mother: We went to [a town nearby], and we had the most horrendous hamburger.
Stepfather: We had a burger, yeah . . .
Question: Right – so why did you have this horrendous beef-burger?
Mother: I hadn't eaten since the morning, since breakfast.
Stepfather: It was about half past three wasn't it?

The 'horrendous hamburger' would not normally be an acceptable part of this woman's food universe at home but on this occasion hunger proved to be an irresistible temptation and resulted in impulse buying.

In the last few paragraphs, then, there is the suggestion that tourists operate according to different rules when eating at home and when eating on holiday. It is, of course, not surprising that there may be different codes of conventions in operation, the one pertaining to life at home and denoted by restraint, the other pertaining to holiday time and denoted by indulgence. Although there are other themes that emerge from the interviews with tourists which deserve extended consideration, it is this on which I focus in the remainder of this chapter.

DIFFERENCES BETWEEN FOOD ON HOLIDAY AND FOOD AT HOME

A little bit of what you fancy does you good.

(Newport retailer)

People on holiday are not interested in healthy eating.

(Newport caterer)

Three T's – they say tasty, tantalising and the other one I forgot what is it . . . tempting I think.

(Newport chef)

A significant number of tourists interviewed claimed there was not much difference between what they ate at home and on holiday, which is unsurprising given the homogeneity fostered by large retail outlets and supermarkets throughout most of the UK. However, this apparent lack of difference between home and holiday eating must be properly contextualised by taking into consideration not only explicit statements by interviewees which qualify the general statement, but also much that may be inferred from detailed information provided about what was eaten at home and on holiday. Much of the latter serves to modify and refine the former claim. In addition to the differences in tempo, pace and time already alluded to, at least four other themes[5] emerge from the data on food on holiday: cooked breakfasts, chips, sweets and puddings, and eating more food than usual, including two- and three-course meals.

The tendency to have a full cooked breakfast while on holiday is a prominent theme in many interviews, in marked contrast to reports of a cup of coffee and a cigarette, a hurried cereal or toast – or even no breakfast at all – at home. While requests to describe breakfasts at home were sometimes greeted by general and loud guffaws of laughter from an entire family, accompanied by the word 'chaos' and conveying a sense of haste, in depicting breakfasts on holiday there are allusions to substantial, long-drawn-out meals, often not finished until well after 10.00 a.m.

Wife: There were a couple of people we sort of got talking to at breakfast time – so our breakfast sort of drew [out] – they were lovely breakfasts, they were really pleasant.
Question: What did you have for breakfast?
Wife: Oh it was lovely breakfast – very full – you could have juice, cereal, fruit, full cooked breakfast and then toast and marmalade and a plentiful supply of coffee and tea – excellent.

The theme of cooked breakfasts on holiday tended to emerge spontaneously from the interviews themselves, as the following examples indicate:

Question: Do you think the food you eat on holiday is very different to the food you eat at home?
Mother: It's slightly different – yes, I mean the pattern of eating, well, isn't as regular . . . we definitely eat more for breakfast because we have much more time . . . on holiday; at home we haven't – we all get up very early because we both commute into London . . . [son's name] is at school in London and I work there so we both commute in so we get up at 6 o'clock and you know, we leave the house at 7.00 and we basically have a piece of toast and get ready for school and get, you know, so on holiday (a) we're all hungrier because we've been taking much more exercise and (b) we've got lots more time. So we're much more inclined to have eggs or bacon or a cooked breakfast of some kind and sit about over it . . .

(Self-caterer)

Question: So you've stayed in bed and breakfasts – have you had hearty breakfasts every day?
Mother: [laughing] Yes!
Daughter: [chuckling] Yes!
Son: Yes.

Question: You have?
Daughter: Yes, full-cooked breakfast every day.
Question: All of you?
Son: Well, not always – a few times –
Father: Yeah – a few times we've just got so full of egg and bacon and sausage and all the rest of it that we've just had to refuse the full cooked breakfast.
Mother: We don't normally eat this you see.
Father: We miss out the egg, or just have scrambled egg on toast or something.
Daughter: Yeah.
Father: But I mean everybody has offered us egg and bacon and sausage and mushrooms.
Daughter: Fried bread.
Father: And tomatoes, fried bread and –
Mother: Tomato juice.
Father: Orange juice, cornflakes and toast thrown in as well.
Question: Right, and do you normally have that at home?
Mother: No.
Daughter: No.
Mother: Definitely not.
Question: No – so what would you have at home?
Son: A bowl of cereal.
Daughter: Yeah, cereal.
Son: And that would be all – maybe a cup of tea. . . .
Father: Yeah – I usually have a bowl of muesli and a cup of tea.
Question: [to mother] And yourself?
Mother: Well, it's either usually toast or grapefruit segments. None of us are really big eaters in the morning, are we?

> (Nuclear family spending their holiday walking the
> 200-mile Pembrokeshire coastal path)

'Bacon and eggs' can, then, be taken as either part of a breakfast or 'brunch' or even eaten any time of the day as a 'fry-up'. This dish thus fits in well with the fact that holiday meals (especially in caravans), like weekend meals, are generally burdened with fewer rules and greater flexibility surrounding their timing. Further, such food is sometimes cooked by the men in the families, and in some cases is one of the few things that men can and do cook, irrespective of social class, as in the following interview:

Question: Do you do most of the cooking and shopping yourself?

Mother: Yeah.

Question: Your husband doesn't cook?

Mother: No – he's just so busy – he goes out in the morning, comes in, you know, and it's time for supper you know.

Question: Yes. Do you find that he sometimes does things at weekends though or on holidays?

Mother: Yes – if he wants to – he'll go and do the bacon, egg, sausages . . . if we're down [in] the caravan – now that would be his ideal breakfast.

Question: And he'll do that himself will he?

Mother: Yeah – yeah – I don't cook it. [laughing]

Question: You don't cook it at all?

Mother: Not very often, no.

Clearly, cooked breakfasts are hugely enjoyed, so much so that sometimes they are an 'ideal breakfast' for some, but they are also seen as a bit taboo and naughty, and therefore regarded as a 'treat' which is to be consumed only rarely. There is a moralistic tinge to some of the remarks made regarding cooked breakfasts, as instanced by two different mothers staying in self-catering caravans, the first stating: 'We do stoop as low as to have bacon and egg on occasions whereas we wouldn't at home normally', and the second stating that she hardly ever had cooked breakfasts either at home or on holiday since: 'I would be a beast if I did.'

If cooked breakfasts arouse ambivalence, chips[6] emerge as an even more highly charged topic in a minority of these interviews. Although considered inferior food, they can also be a 'treat'. It is striking that in three interviews, middle-class mothers expressed a strong moral interdiction against chips:

Mother: There is something else I've immediately realised we eat when we go out here that we never eat at home – we virtually never have chips at home – we've eliminated them from the diet really, except on the very occasional occasion like when my son said to me a couple of years ago, well, rather movingly one night, 'Why aren't we like normal families?' and I thought 'Oh my God, what's coming now?' you know – and I said, 'How so? What are we not normal in?' [and he replied] 'Why don't we just have hamburgers and chips for dinner?' So we have oven chips for him two or three times a year but otherwise we never have chips at home. Does anyone have a chip pan any more? But when we go out here we often have chips – I often have a jacket potato but even I have chips sometimes and my son has chips a lot and my husband has chips quite a lot.

Mothers who monitor their children's food intake are acting in what they consider to be the children's best interests but against the children's possible opposition and in the three interviews concerned the topic emerged as a source of possible conflict and negotiation within families. However, what is considered unacceptable within the home is more acceptable outside where, in any case, children's actions often cannot be so closely monitored or controlled by the parents, and is dependent on what is available in public places. All children, as one interviewee observed, tend to love chips, and on holidays mothers tend to be more indulgent:

> *Question*: Can I ask you, because you've got children, what your view of chips is?
> *Woman*: I like them but we have them once maybe twice a week, but no more than that, so it's not chips with everything.
> *Question*: Is there a difference between holidays and home?
> *Woman*: Oh yeah.
> *Question*: And what's the difference?
> *Woman*: Well the difference is that you're relaxed, you're not going to say: 'Right you will sit down and you will eat this, this and this', you'll say: 'Right what do you want, there you are, sit down and eat it.'
> *Question*: And you let them have what they want?
> *Woman*: Within reason.

In over half of the interviews there is explicit evidence that more of these food items are consumed on holiday than at home. Interestingly, the presence of the same moral interdiction in these statements coexists with vastly differing standards of what is an acceptable frequency with which chips are eaten at home. One mother claimed that at home: 'We don't have an awful lot of chips', specifying only about once a fortnight, while another mother in a family which had adopted a 'conscious healthy eating policy' with strict limits on the consumption of sugar, stated: 'We try and limit chips to about twice a week at home, whereas perhaps on holiday one tends to have something with chips', and a third mother claimed they 'never had chips at home' and that they had them when out only occasionally. By contrast with other interviewees, only one informant ate far more chips at home than he did on holiday. A self-defined working-class man, he acknowledged unabashedly that: 'I'm afraid I'm a chip and butty man' and that he sometimes had chips 'twice of an evening' at home, whereas on holiday in Newport he and his relatives were eating most evenings in a restaurant of good reputation where no chips had been served on principle for years.

The overall conclusion drawn from the data presented so far is that there is a greater indulgence in cooked breakfasts and fish and chips on holiday and that behaviour surrounding these foodstuffs is characterised by greater restraint at home. A fortiori, there is a common association between being on holiday and 'treating' onself. This theme of 'treats' can embrace a whole repertoire of foodstuffs from haute cuisine to cream cakes:

> *Daughter*: Unfortunately I had the biggest cream tea I've ever seen in my life which [my brother and sister present at interview] shared with me.
> *Son*: Aah – Aah!
> *Question*: [laughing] Well, is that something you would do at home?
> *Daughter*: No, I don't eat cakes normally.
> *Question*: I mean is it something that you do on breaks? Do you tend to be more lax on breaks, because you're away from home?
> *Mother*: I do.
> *Question*: What did you have on Sunday?
> *Stepfather*: Too much. Sunday was an odd day because – we were talking about it actually – because we had [cooked] breakfast here [at pub/hotel dining room], we had lunch at a hotel, which was a traditional sort of Sunday roast, and then we ate again back here [at pub/hotel dining room] that night. ...We were only saying actually that we would *never* eat like this at home – three cooked meals in a day, but then – you know – we're out walking – we play golf – you know – and you get hungry, you get peckish, especially when someone else is cooking it.

Reports of the relaxation of 'restraints' normally in operation and 'enjoying' treats on holiday – as well as the theme of eating more – is often accompanied by a laughter which is indicative of ambivalence: guilt and enjoyment of items that are clearly 'naughty and nice', and a contradiction between food that is enjoyable (on holiday) and food that is healthy (at home).

HEALTHY EATING AND COMPETING PARADIGMS OF HEALTH

In previous sections I have provided substantial evidence to demonstrate the existence of an ethic of release and relaxation on holidays in relation to food. It is arguable that contemporary British citizens, like contemporary Americans, 'are the objects and subjects of two opposing mandates, two opposing approaches to achieve well-being' (Crawford 1984: 92). At the level of the social system this structural opposition is a principal contradiction. The culture of consumption demands a modal personality contrary to that required for production. The mandate for discipline clashes with the mandate for pleasure; symbols of self-control and discipline associated with the work ethic (the week/at home) contradict the symbols of release from those controls (the weekend/holidays). The contradiction in structure leads to a conflict in experience so that, for instance, one must consume and stay thin at the same time; after and even before holidays one must diet.

> *Question*: So you've been here a whole week. Have you tended to eat something outside the home that you wouldn't normally eat at home?
> *Answer*: We don't diet when we're on holiday.
> *Question*: You don't diet – do you normally diet?
> *Answer*: Yes – a lot – it usually lasts two days before I lapse.

On being asked about healthy eating the majority of tourists were aware of current advice and most, though not all, had changed their diets in some way as a result. Thus a mother noted that her notion of a 'good mix of food' involved 'not too much red meat, less fat, a lot of fresh fruit and veg'. Some other interviewees, however, stated that they thought food should be enjoyed or that they ate what they wanted, did not take much notice of healthy eating advice and did not let it 'worry' them. Some said they did not consciously try to eat healthily although they believed they were so doing. By contrast to health as self-control, health as release is epitomised by enjoyment, relaxation: 'a little bit of what you fancy does you good'. It is the modality of 'health as self-control' with which 'healthy eating' is resisted by the male in the following interview, in contrast to his wife:

Question: Do you think diet affects health?
Wife: Yes.
Question: So what steps do you take? I mean all this advice about health and eating?
Wife: I'm very good at giving advice [laughing] . . .
Husband: I don't believe any of it.
Wife: and very poor at taking it. Um, I mean, I am over-weight . . .
Husband: Oh I don't like decaff. I eat real butter and all that sort of stuff. Don't pay a lot of attention to . . .
Wife: Well, I mean it does influence me. You see these things, you hear it, I mean the scare about . . .
Husband: If you believed everything that you read and you heard you wouldn't eat or drink anything. I like best butter, I've never changed from best butter. Don't like margarine, best butter to me is natural. And I like best butter, yeah? And I like meat, red meat, white meat, any meat. And I do – I don't mind fruit. But I like natural things – I'm not into beefburgers and these bloody things.

As Crawford points out, the existence of two opposing models – such as control and release – is rarely a tidy affair. One way of reconciling the opposing themes of control and release is through the notion of 'balance', which is a third symbolic modality which has been noted by a number of authors (Fischler 1986, Backett *et al.* 1994, Keane and Willetts 1995). Crawford notes in his article:

The new health consciousness belongs to neither control nor release. People often speak of the necessity for 'balance' or the avoidance of 'extremes'. And certainly, each symbol and its corresponding experiences find their power in opposition, an opposition that is perhaps basic to human life. The specific content of these forms, however, a product of living cultures, raises questions as to their easy integration. The contemporary mandates for control and release, reflecting a basic contra-diction in the social body, mitigate against such a balance. The pursuit of health is bound to reproduce that contradiction.

(1984: 94)

Again and again in these interviews with tourists in Wales the notion of balance, 'everything in moderation', finding a 'happy medium' and a varied diet is paramount in response to explicit questions on healthy eating (though what people mean by a 'balanced diet' varies considerably).

In everyday life, nonetheless, as the interviews conducted here indicate, some people tend to adopt one, some another, while many juggle both. Another way of reconciling such contradictions may be achieved through separate contexts of time and place, and from the evidence presented here, it is clear that for most people, holiday time, in a holiday resort, means that 'release' modalities are not only operationalised, but also sanctioned. Part of 'balance', then, is the contrast between work and leisure, separated in time and space, each of which has its own ethic symbolised by food.

NOTES

1 These figures were obtained from the Welsh Tourist Office in Cardiff, those for the UK being provisional.
2 Food on holiday constituted one of the issues I investigated whilst working on the 'Concepts of Healthy Eating' project based at the Department of Anthropology, Goldsmiths' College and directed by Professor Pat Caplan. It was part of a larger research programme 'The Nation's Diet: The Social Science of Food Choice', funded by the Economic and Social Research Programme and directed by Professor Anne Murcott.
3 In 1990 second-home ownership reached 24 per cent (about one in four) of local homes in Newport (Carningli Rural Initiative 1994: 19).
4 Whereas formerly pubs relied on the sale of drinks and alcohol as their main income, nowadays the sale of food is essential to economic survival.
5 Other themes which emerged from interview data was a tendency by some to choose more elaborate dishes whilst eating out than they might want to prepare at home, to choose items which were not liked by other family members, to choose shellfish and seafood, to look for local and Welsh items, and a greater indulgence in alcohol on holiday.
6 At the time of field-work, Newport itself had not had a fish and chip shop for many years, although a van visited the town regularly on Friday evenings throughout the year.

REFERENCES

Backett, K., Davison, C. and Mullen, K. (1994) 'Lay evaluation of health and healthy life-styles: evidence from three studies', *British Journal of General Practice* 44: 277–80.

Carningli Rural Initiative (1994) [1991] *Draft Action Plan for Newport*, Newport, Pembs.

Crawford, Robert (1984) 'A cultural account of "health": control, release and the social body', in J.B. McKinlay (ed.) *Issues in the Political Economy of Health Care*, New York: Tavistock.

Douglas, Mary (1966) *Purity and Danger: An Analysis of Concepts of Pollution and Taboo*, London: Routledge and Kegan Paul.

—— (1970) *Natural Symbols: Explorations in Cosmology*, New York: Pantheon.

Fischler, C. (1986) 'Learned versus "spontaneous" dietetics: French mothers' views of what children should eat', *Social Science Information* 25, 4: 945–65.

Foucault, M. (1978) *The History of Sexuality: An Introduction*, New York: Pantheon.

Keane, A. and Willetts, A. (1995) 'Concepts of healthy eating: an anthropological investigation in South-East London', Working Paper (mimeo), London: Goldsmiths' College.

Turner, T. (1980) 'The social skin: bodily adornment, social meaning and personal identity', in J. Cherfas and R. Lewin (eds) *Not Working Alone*, London: Temple Smith.

Chapter 9

Too hard to swallow?

The palatability of healthy eating advice

Anne Keane

Information about food and health is a key contemporary issue. National campaigns to reduce the incidence of obesity and dietary-related diseases have met with little success, while in recent years the role of government departments, food producers, manufacturers and retailers has come under increasing public scrutiny in relation to food safety issues.

Qualitative research into food practices often concentrates on abstract symbolic meanings rather than considering broader historical and political processes. In contrast, literature dealing with food consumption in terms of economics or policy rarely considers the complexity of people's behaviour. The aim of this paper is to avoid such a division, by discussing both the results of a qualitative study into perceptions of food and health information and the wider political and commercial context of such information.[1]

SETTING THE SCENE: THE HISTORICAL CONTEXT OF HEALTHY EATING

Throughout this century the government has conceptualised dietary change as a consumer issue, rather than a state or industry responsibility. Concerns about the healthiness of the British diet have, however, shifted significantly during this period. In the early 1900s attention was focused on malnutrition among the working classes, and the accompanying threat to industrial productivity and the nation's capacity to defend itself. Resulting from the development of nutritional theories during the first half of the century, foods with a high protein and vitamin content were classified as 'protective' and calorific foods such as cereals, bread, rice and sugar as 'energy bearing' (Cannon 1992). Healthy eating was largely to do with achieving and maintaining 'strength'. However, since the 1970s attention has shifted to the so-called 'diseases of affluence': chronic diseases, particularly cardiovascular diseases, cancer and diabetes, which have been linked to diets high in fat, sugar and salt, and low in fibre.

Mills's (1992) historical review of food policy demonstrates that the British state's prime concern throughout this century has been the security of food supply. The government has been unwilling to intervene directly in food production in order to achieve health-related dietary changes for the population unless such nutritional concerns have been in harmony with the interests of the food producers and industry. For example the state's encouragement of milk production during the inter-war period was not primarily due to concern about health (milk was regarded as one of the superior 'protective' foods) but the result of a rare 'coincidence of interests between milk producers and consumers' (Mills 1992: 80). State intervention targeted only particular vulnerable groups such as children and expectant mothers. Despite widespread malnutrition among the working classes, general measures to improve diets as a whole were not part of the government's agenda.

Nutritional expertise was primarily employed by the government on a problem-solving basis, such as during war-time, rather than in relation to long-term planning. Rationing during the Second World War included an element of health and welfare policy: for example, intake of iron and B vitamins was increased by raising the wheatmeal content of bread.[2] After the war, government priorities were geared to the maximisation of food production, and a corresponding close relationship between the Ministry of Agriculture Fisheries and Food (MAFF)[3] and the National Farmers Union (NFU) was established. During the 1940s and 1950s and the post-war reconstruction of Britain, 'cheap sources of calories were identified as vital national resources' (Cannon 1992: 21). Food production focused on hard fats and processed sugars with the processed food industry profiting considerably from government policies.

The assumptions of the 1950s about lasting improvements in the standard of living as part and parcel of the consumer society proved to be unfounded. Concern about the nation's diet resurfaced in the 1970s along with increasing poverty for certain sectors of the population. A number of chronic diseases began to be linked to diet through epidemiological cross-cultural comparison and migrant studies.

The political implications of nutrition policies became matters of media and public attention during the early 1980s when the government's reluctance to intervene in the market freedom of the food industry became evident in relation to the publication of the NACNE report. The government had set up the National Advisory Council on Nutrition Education (NACNE) in 1979 to report and advise on the growing international body of research linking diet with disease. A working party of doctors and nutritionists was appointed to report on the constitution of a healthy diet. Theirs was the first British report to recommend quantified reductions in the consumption of fat, sugar and salt and an increase in fibre consumption, although similar documents had been previously published in other industrialised countries. The report worked on the premise that the whole population was 'at risk' from dietary related diseases which had clear implications for policy changes. Representatives on NACNE from MAFF, the Department of Health and Social Security, and the food industry, objected to the first three drafts of the report (Cannon 1987). A draft report was leaked to the press in 1983. The report was eventually published, but as a 'discussion document' for health professionals rather than an official government publication (Cannon 1987).

The Committee on Medical Aspects of Food Policy (COMA) report on diet and cardiovascular disease in 1984 was the official response to controversy over the NACNE report. However, the COMA report only gave targets for fats and saturated fats, not for sugar and salt. Recommended changes affecting the food industry were also much diluted in subsequent policy. For example, the introduction of nutritional labelling was done in a way that allowed all sectors of industry 'the opportunity to present information which is favourable to their products' (Mills 1992: 143).

Despite the persistence of the close relationship between MAFF and the food industry, important changes in the 'food policy community' started during the 1970s (Smith 1991). As a result of the UK's membership of the European Community, farmers' and manufacturers' interests began to diverge. In addition, manufacturers and retailers began to pursue different strategies, establishing their own separate information and lobbying groups. Consumer and medical groups became increasingly vocal on issues of food quality and food policy during the 1980s.[4] The salmonella crisis of

1988, which divided MAFF and the Department of Health (DoH), made it clear that there was no longer one single governmental decision-making centre regarding food policy (Smith 1991, Miller and Reilly 1994a). Equally, since this incident 'the increased number of groups involved in food issues and the interest of the media means that the government is finding it much more difficult to manage food policy' (Smith 1991: 252).

RECENT CONTEXT

The perceived necessity to limit the costs of state health care has formed an increasingly significant element of government rhetoric during the 1980s and 1990s. Current health policy stresses that 'everyone has a part to play' in attaining health targets for the population (Department of Health 1992: 5), and points to the need for 'healthy alliances' between the government, public sector organisations, the NHS, voluntary groups and employers. The notion that health education can enable people to 'make informed decisions about their health and that of their families' (Department of Health 1992: 36) is also reiterated. For diet and nutrition, the targets include reducing the average percentage of food energy derived by the population from saturated fatty acids and total fats, and reducing the percentages of men and women who are obese,[5] by the year 2005. To date there has been little or no progress towards the dietary targets, in fact the incidence of obesity is continuing to rise (Department of Health 1995). An estimated 20 million British adults are overweight, 6 million of whom are obese (West 1994).

In the summer of 1994 the confectionery and snack sectors of the food industry became worried that the forthcoming COMA report on diet and cardiovascular disease, would contain much more specific dietary recommendations than given in the *Health of the Nation* document. Already large donors to the Conservative Party, a number of companies increased their lobbying activities. The subsequent leaking of COMA's draft discussion document to the press in August allowed the food industry's publicity machine the opportunity to rubbish the report's recommendations prior to its official publication in November. The views of food industry spokespersons that the recommendations constituted unnecessary government interference, and could potentially lead to massive job losses in the food industry, were widely publicised in the media.

The food industry also claimed that the scientific basis of the report was unproven on the basis that sugar and salt were not risk factors in cardiovascular disease. In response to previous criticisms that nutritional information generally contained little practical advice in terms of foods, the new COMA report gave specific recommendations about how many portions of a range of foods should be consumed each day or week to reduce the risk of heart disease. The report also recommended a reduction in salt consumption, which had not been mentioned in the 'Health of the Nation' policy. When the report was published some government health spokespersons emphasised that, in fact, the report was not part of government policy, and that the recommendations were aimed at the level of the population as a whole rather than at individuals, thus rather diluting its significance.

The Nutrition Task Force (established as part of the 'Health of the Nation' policy to formulate action plans to reach the dietary targets) made little progress in those areas which affected the food industry before it was disbanded in October 1995. For example, schemes to develop graphical nutritional labelling were abandoned and plans to establish targets for the reduction of fat and salt in processed foods also had little support from the food industry (National Food Alliance, Autumn 1995: 1, see also Department of Health 1996).

Throughout this century, then, the government's commitment to promoting healthy eating policies has clearly been shaped by the interests of the food industry and the responsibility for healthy eating has been placed on the consumer. The development of the institutional separation between food and health issues throughout this period, with a *laissez-faire* attitude to the market place, is central to the debates about the location of responsibility for national dietary problems.

RESPONSIBILITY, HEALTH PROMOTION AND INFORMATION

The concept of health *promotion* superseded that of health education during the 1970s. According to its advocates this new approach actively promoted 'health' rather than simply the prevention of illness, and represented a significant shift from earlier individual-istic heath education towards a new emphasis on empowerment and community-based strategies. In reality, new health promotion models often retained the importance of educating individuals to make informed health choices. The notion of rational actors, utilising knowledge to change their attitudes and thus alter their behaviour, continued to dominate policy (Lupton 1995).

Health promotion models have been significantly challenged by those calling for a more social understanding of health and illness and the recognition of material limitations to 'choice'. For example Davison et al. (1991) argue that, in standard health promotion discourse, political issues concerning the relationship between the individual and social responsibility are cast as 'an essentially unproblematical relationship between knowledge (the awareness of information) and the decision to do healthy things (or not do healthy things)' (1991: 3). Health promotion material has also been criticised for not taking its audience needs into account, for simplifying issues of probability and risk and for a lack of adequate targeting of health advice (Farrant and Russell 1986, Wilson 1989). The macro context of poor nutrition, and the practical and financial impossibilities of eating healthily for certain sectors of the population are regularly reiterated by research on poverty and diet (Cole-Hamilton and Lang 1986, Lobstein 1991, National Children's Home 1991, Leather 1992, Dobson et al. 1994). Problems for those on low incomes include lack of access to cheaper food retailers, an inability to buy in bulk and therefore save money, less margin for experimentation and limited cooking facilities. Money set aside for food tends to be the most elastic part of the household budget.

The contextualisation of health practices is a key theoretical issue with repercussions for debates about individual 'freedom of choice'. Although the critique of an individualistic and 'victim-blaming' approach to health education is well established, recently social scientists have argued that academic research often compounds the problem by reifying 'health beliefs' as part of a realm which exists apart from everyday life. This approach tends to maintain an unhelpful conceptual division between 'belief' and 'behaviour' (Williams 1995). Backett (1992), for example, argues that the individualistic orientation of much research has been detrimental to an adequate understanding of the contexts within which individuals operate. Taking the household as the unit of analysis, she comments that: 'health-relevant behaviours have to be seen as one aspect of prioritising and decision making about time allocation in daily life' (Backett 1992: 267).

A necessary corollary to the 'lifestyle' approach to dietary change implicit in health promotion models is the provision of adequate and accurate information for individuals to make informed choices. As shown by the discussion of previous policy, the translation of scientific research into health promotion materials is a highly politicised process. Furthermore, debates about the lack of public adherence to healthy eating advice often concentrate on officially sponsored campaigns and thus tend to ignore the variety of information sources concerning food and health. In reality, such information comes from a diverse range of sources which do not all give the same message or have the same intention. Fine and Wright (1991) discuss the failings of current health education models which are based on the concept of the 'trickle down' of nutritional information. The assumption that information decides food choice ignores the fact that consumers cannot determine which foods are available in the food system. It also neglects the existence of diverse informal sources of knowledge including retailing practices and advertising.

In a very competitive market, creating new 'healthy' foods or, more often, 'healthier' versions of popular foods is one strategy to increase market share. Thus the quantity of foods available has increased, rather than 'unhealthier' food products being replaced. Recently, a new trend in 'functional foods' has become evident; these are foods claiming special health benefits, such as lowering cholesterol, on the basis of specific ingredients. More generally, products are often misleadingly promoted on the selective high-lighting of supposed health qualities, for example, concentrating on one aspect of a product such as 'low in fat', but neglecting to also mention 'high in sugar'. Indeed, Longfield (1992) argues that packaging and labelling have to be seen as part of advertising because they establish and maintain the image of a product.

The weight-loss industry has also co-opted the discourse of 'healthy eating' to sell its often unhealthy products. This multi-million industry thrives on the fact that diets are rarely successful: studies regularly show that only a minority of dieters (usually around 5 per cent) manage to maintain their weight loss for a significant length of time, and the majority usually gain more weight in the long term (Garner and Wooley 1991). The market for meal replacement products (such as 'slimming' drinks and biscuits) alone is estimated at £20 million per year. Many of these products are in fact high in sugar and fats and not significantly lower in calories than comparable non-slimming products; they are also more expensive (Dibb 1992).

A simplistic view of food and health information neglects the massive resources which the food industry and retailers have at their disposal in comparison to publicly funded health promotion services. The money spent by the Health Education Authority (HEA) on nutrition education is insignificant compared to that spent on food advertising. For example, the HEA received £700,000 funding specifically for nutrition education for 1996–7 (personal communication, Department of Health 1996), while in 1995, £551 million was spent on food and drink advertising (personal communication, Advertising Association 1996). Confectionery is the most heavily advertised food category followed by coffee, fast foods and soft drinks (Longfield 1992). The majority of advertisements on children's television are for food and drinks; breakfast cereals are the most heavily advertised, followed by confectionery, fast foods, soft drinks, ice-cream and lollies (Food Commission 1994). As well as explicit advertising, many food manufacturers and trade organisations now produce their own 'information' material about food and health which they distribute to schools and health authorities. Typically, commercially produced leaflets tend to concentrate on brand products and give nutritional information primarily with product emphasis (Lobstein 1990: 22–3). Recent years have seen an increasing number of joint ventures between the public and private sectors, with the Health Education Authority logo appearing on a range of commercially produced material.

In summary, healthy eating is clearly a political issue and the majority of 'information' about food and health is driven by commercial considerations, particularly in terms of advertising and product descriptions and, more implicitly, by the government's reluctance to intervene in the 'freedom' of the market. This reluctance to intervene is in contrast to highly interventionist policies pursued in relation to food production, particularly since the introduction of the Common Agricultural Policy. The unwillingness to legislate on the quality of information provided by the food industry clearly limits the possibility of accurate information being made available to the public. As can be seen in the following section, participants in this study were clearly sceptical of the links between government and industry.

ETHNOGRAPHIC DATA

The remainder of this paper explores how people use and value healthy eating information, using data from a wide-ranging qualitative study of contemporary ideas about food and health in South-East London. Field-work was carried out between October 1993 and September 1994. Participants in the study included women and men who came from a range of age and class backgrounds, the predominant ethnic backgrounds being white British and black British of Afro-Caribbean origin. Data from 134 in-depth semi-structured participant interviews will be discussed here, along with data from interviews with local health professionals.

Obtaining information

Participants obtained information about food and health from a diverse range of sources including 'the media', friends and relatives, official health education material, supermarket leaflets, books, specialist organisations and health professionals. Information about healthy eating was perceived to be generally 'around' and participants often found it difficult to identify from which source and at what time they had come to 'know' particular examples of information which they quoted as fact. Acquiring knowledge about healthy eating was often described as a process of osmosis which did not require much attention: 'I think I do take in a lot of things that are around me but I don't really think about it consciously, I just sort of store it' (Woman aged 24). It was also felt that information about what to eat or rather what not to eat was hard to avoid: 'You can't help but be aware of it, these days.' Many reported that they had reached saturation point concerning information about food and health, and thus tended to ignore new advice.

The necessity to obtain new information about food and health was seen as time-specific and was related to particular stages in the life-cycle. Typical times for women were during pregnancy or when bringing up young children, while men became more interested in healthy eating information in their 40s and 50s, when they had reached a publicly recognised 'at risk' age for a heart attack. Young men in their 20s often expressed a blasé attitude to future health problems, while participants in their 60s and older felt there was little to be gained by changing their diet, unless they had a specific health problem.

The majority of participants characterised food and health information as contradictory and changing 'all the time': 'One day zinc is good for you the next it's bad. It's a minefield. No one could possibly be expected to understand all of it' (Man aged 37). Changes in advice were seen as 'proof' that information generally was worthless, rather than as resulting from scientific advances. The existence of conflicting advice meant it was impossible to judge what one should eat and what one should avoid on the basis of external information alone. Some participants, predominantly middle-class, elaborated their arguments along the lines that there were bound to be contradictions in advice, because the relationship between food and health was complicated. The example of cholesterol was frequently cited as evidence of contradictions: 'They were convinced that cholesterol-high foods were very bad for us until very recently and now they all seem to be going the other way, some cholesterol-rich foods are actually good' (Woman aged 43). Participants explained their lack of faith in new information in terms of the absence of definitive scientific proof about how foods could affect health. They felt that the variability of individual responses to food and diet made general predictions of 'risk' of little relevance.

Relevance of information and assessments of risk

Participants did not regard general information concerning a healthy diet as applicable to their own situations. People saw not being ill as proof that they were eating well and therefore any new information was deemed irrelevant. The majority of participants felt that eating a healthy diet strengthened the body's 'defences' against minor illnesses: 'If you eat a good diet, you're less likely to give in to some bug' (Man aged 34). They judged the healthiness of their diet in terms of how much general 'energy' they had and how often they experienced minor illnesses such as colds and flu. Participants' own *embodied knowledge*, i.e. how patterns of food consumption affected them personally, was therefore crucial to their understanding of the relationship between food and health. While very aware of the association between high fat consumption and heart disease, participants were often reluctant to comment on something of which they had no personal experience. It was acknowledged that *in principle* certain diets could have a positive effect on health but commonly participants would qualify a general statement about diet because they felt that it was not possible to generalise. Worrying about potential illnesses in the future was felt to be counterproductive, although participants did look for dietary information when they were ill.

Embodied knowledge interacted with other sources. The information that participants had gained through their own observations and discussions with others was also part of their understanding of disease aetiology. Davison *et al.* (1992) describe this as 'lay epidemiology'. Participants regarded general healthy eating advice as simplistic and inadequate because it did not portray the complexities of disease causation, particularly the fact that some people are more susceptible to heart disease than others. Genetic or environmental factors were often regarded as more influential than individual behaviour.

Participants in their 20s and 30s were more likely to stress the importance of heredity in dictating one's own susceptibility to illness than those in other age groups. As one 24-year-old woman explained:

> Do you know the honest truth, [healthy eating] is a hit and miss situation. You've got some people who have eaten healthy foods all their lives and still end up with coronary disease and you've got people who eat all these fats and stuff and never get it. It depends on the person's family background first of all, you have to take into consideration that certain things happen in certain families.

Many participants in this age group felt that this individual variability was a valid reason for not making dietary changes with the aim of preventing illness. Although they had often made some health-related dietary changes, their concerns about healthy eating were explained in terms of how they felt now, rather than with reference to their future. Indeed there was a generalised perception that it was counterproductive to 'think too much' about one's diet.

Older participants were more likely to refer to unspecified predispositions to illness, than to genetics or family background: 'If you're susceptible to it, it's unfortunate if you're the one, but it's going to happen to you no matter what you do' (Woman aged 45). The random aspect of illness meant that it was pointless to worry about how one could prevent it. Participants in their 60s and older often expressed this quite forcibly:

It's important once you know you've got an illness to treat it accordingly but you can't surely spend the whole of your life concentrating so much on what's going to make you ill, because you don't know what's going to make you ill.

(Woman aged 69)

Participants who did make changes based on the principle of preventing dietary-related disease were usually in the 40–60 year age-range and tended to be white and middle class. Men, particularly, often sought new information about food and health when they perceived themselves as having reached a vulnerable age for heart attacks. Age was not such a significant factor in increasing women's awareness of healthy eating. Women tended to be much more aware of food and health information throughout their lives due to being more consistently concerned about their responsibility for their family's health and, more generally, irrespective of family situation, because of concerns about their weight and appearance. Food and health issues were widely perceived as part of a feminine rather than masculine remit. Men often described dietary changes, such as reducing fat intake, as part of their female partner's agenda rather than their own, or put such changes in the context of family relationships or their conventionally masculine role as 'provider' for the family, rather than in terms of their own health or subjectivity. One man explained that he had made changes because he had got married: 'It seemed the sensible thing to do, particularly since kids are on the agenda, to have a medical check up and to take at least some precautions.' However, dietary changes at this age were by no means universal. A 46-year-old man, aware of his impending 'old age', was adamant that he wasn't going to give up his enjoyment of food:

I'm starting to perceive my own mortality a lot more directly. I'm getting quite close to 50 now. I don't feel it but I know that it is happening. I can see my body falling apart and I can see the end of life coming and I'm unhappy about that and to some extent I think I ought to be thinking about my diet, I ought to be doing the exercise, I ought to be doing that, I don't of course.

Scepticism about information sources

Commonly information was described as coming from a general 'they' which included scientists, the medical profession, journalists and promoters of new diets. This tendency to homogenise information sources was indicative of the perception that advice about health emanated from distant but interfering external sources which had little understanding of 'real life', in which things were complicated and to which generalising theories could not be applied.

There was clear scepticism concerning governmental and commercial sources of information. Many participants maintained that it was necessary to treat all information with suspicion and reported that they judged information according to its source and who was likely to benefit from it. They felt that there was no reliable external source of advice about food and health and saw themselves as keeping an independent and 'healthy' distance from 'expert' advice. As a 31-year-old woman explained, her own experience was more constant and reliable:

> I tend not to believe any of it really, I think that food research is often financed by people who have an interest in a certain outcome. So I find it very difficult to take any of that seriously. But obviously I think that certain things just must be healthier, you know, common sense tells me that eating good fresh food is.

Generalising information was thus criticised for being based on political and commercial considerations. It was felt that information did not arise from a concern for the public's health but was primarily a marketing strategy on the part of food manufacturers and retailers. Some described the interests of the government and the food industry as synonymous – part of a corrupt 'establishment'. As one woman said, referring to BSE:[6] 'You've got to use your own judgement, someone else will come along and say the opposite to them, so with the beef thing the government are going to say something different because they want you to buy it don't they?' (Woman aged 27). Distrust of the relationship between government and the food industry was clearest in respect of people's concerns about the health effects of modern food production methods and food processing. There was a feeling that *real* information about food and health was being hidden from the public. Participants felt that there was enough material telling them what *they* should do about healthy eating but there was a lack of accurate information about larger food production processes which could potentially cause ill health. Mothers of young children in particular expressed much concern about additives, and those on a low budget felt that they were unable to afford 'natural' and healthier foods for their children because of their cost in comparison to cheaper, processed foods.

Some participants explained that the lack of 'real' information was a valid reason for not modifying their own consumption to correspond to healthy eating advice, because the effects of making dietary changes could only be negligible compared to all the harmful effects which they *did not* know about. As one 35-year-old man said: 'It's a bit of a farce really when people try and control their diets, because you've got all these hidden additives in food which means you just don't know what you're eating.' Those who had tried to find out about additives had found it very difficult to obtain information which they could use in a practical way, as one 64-year-old woman remarked:

> You read the labels, but that's another thing, you don't always know what they mean. They give you all these E numbers [but] you've got to look it up in your little book and see what E240 means. I mean it doesn't mean anything to you and even if they did give you the name of it, it wouldn't convey anything to me because I'm not a chemist. You have to be really well up in chemistry and things like that to know what it is.

The media were also commonly described as an unreliable source of information. Participants were more likely to stress their scepticism of the media than to credit it as a source of information that affected them personally, although documentaries had more of an impact than news features. Participants were very dismissive of 'sensationalist' reporting, often to the extent that they questioned whether some media coverage contained any factual basis at all. Participants singled out the media's role in 'intensifying' food 'scares', in addition to what they generally perceived as simplistic reporting of food and health issues and the short-lived nature of news coverage. Concentration of media coverage on specific foods, as opposed to the whole diet, was discounted as alarmist and counter to the general healthy eating principles of balance, variety and moderation. Many participants felt that media coverage rarely told them anything new, rather it just reinforced their existing knowledge, particularly the importance of 'moderation' (cf. Lupton and Chapman 1995).

Although participants asserted their scepticism of 'the media', this did not preclude them having made changes to their consumption patterns prompted by something they had read, listened to on the radio or seen on television. Such changes were made on an *ad hoc* basis and depended on what participants felt was relevant to them at that particular time. Dietary changes based on information from the media usually involved increasing consumption of foods or supplements which would potentially *maximise* health, rather than cutting out elements of the diet that were potentially *harmful* to health in the long term.[7] Furthermore, such changes in consumption were often short-lived:

> I enjoy reading that sort of stuff which describes Italians and how they eat olive oil and how nobody gets fat because olive oil is good for you especially if you eat it with tomatoes or whatever it is, stuff like that. I'll think, that's quite interesting and I'll go for that and I may well eat tomatoes and olive oil for the following week or so.
>
> (Man, 34 years old)

In contrast to general participants, many health professionals in the study felt that the media did have a big influence on people's eating habits and regarded it as something which they had to fight against to get their message across. Most health professionals felt that the media tended to concentrate on particular 'scare' stories, creating an unhelpful climate for public awareness of basic healthy eating principles. Many criticised the media's promotion of slimness as the ideal for women. The health professionals' inclusion of advertising within their reference to 'the media' was in contrast to other participants, who typically referred to the media in terms of newspaper articles, radio programmes and television programmes and did not regard advertising as a source of information. Most participants dismissed the notion that they could be affected by advertisements, although they were often concerned about advertising in relation to children.

Health professionals as information sources

Health professionals were important sources of information for participants in relation to specific issues such as advice about feeding young children, although participants rarely went to health professionals for advice unless they had a particular health problem. Age was a significant factor in attitudes towards GPs.

Older participants were more likely to perceive their GP as a source of factual and authoritative advice, in contrast to younger participants for whom GPs had no special status in comparison with other sources of information. Some had found that in their own experience health professionals had been unhelpful on the subject of diet. As one 23-year-old said: 'I don't really trust doctors and nutritionists 'cos they tend to contradict themselves.' Generally, younger participants were much more likely to 'shop around' for information rather than rely on one source.

Information from personal experience

Often critical of 'expert' and official sources of information, participants identified their own personal experience and knowledge as the most reliable and enduring basis of knowledge about food and their own health. One constant theme in participants' discussion of healthy eating information, regardless of age, gender, class or ethnicity, was their own *individuality*. Generalising pronouncements about food and health did not take account of individual differences and therefore did not apply to them. People had a strong belief in learning by their own experience. On the wide spectrum of assertions of individuality, the two polarised positions were: (a) personal independence based on one's food preferences and (b) personal independence based on knowledge of one's own body. These were associated with some age, gender and class differences.

A predominantly older male and/or working-class discourse was a stated lack of concern for authority and their own independence as opposed to others who followed things blindly: 'Someone else might take notice of it but it doesn't affect me really' (Man aged 62 years). Middle-class and female participants were more likely to refer to a knowledge of their own bodies that they had acquired over time: 'I'm still convinced about roughage and refined food and sugar for instance. I feel quite anti-sugar. I am sure it must be bad for you, because I can see, you know, the way sugar affects me' (Woman aged 34 years). Women also tended to draw on a greater variety of discourses about food and health than men.

Older participants often reported that the information about food which they had received from their mothers or what they had had to eat when they were growing up, was all they needed to know about eating healthily. The principles of variety, balance and moderation, which participants attributed to learning in childhood, were the key to assessing if new information was useful or merely 'faddy'. In practical terms 'balance' was not a harmonious overall pattern of consumption but more often a process of trade-offs between 'good' and 'bad' consumption patterns or foods. Balance also referred to balancing health concerns with other day-to-day priorities (see Backett 1992). Among younger participants there was often greater recognition that ideas about health had altered since the previous generation. Younger middle-class participants were more likely than other participants to experiment with their diets, although they still emphasised the importance of balance, variety and moderation. Information about food and health was also transmitted upwards between generations by younger participants to their parents.

Information from friends or relatives often had more of an impact on participants' consumption patterns than more formalised advice. The importance of this informal network has often been neglected in previous literature which has focused primarily on how official information impacts on the public or on highlighting the differences between 'lay' and medical definitions. Sometimes participants validated this kind of information with reference to their friends' or relatives' specialised knowledge or particular interest in food and health issues. However, more generally the value of the informal network was that it was based on the exchange of information – a dialogue about specifics, rather than simply advice 'from above' based on abstract physiological or general principles. Such information was often derived from personal experience, which was regarded as the most authentic source. Discussions with friends or relatives also tended to be more relevant to the day-to-day practicalities of shopping and preparing food. Informal networks were particularly important for women, for whom food was often a topic of general conversation, whereas informal discussions about food and health for men were more strictly confined to specific contexts of sport or exercise activities where discussions of the body and health were deemed appropriate.

Informal networks were not simply sources of novel advice or information but were forums in which other sources of information such as television programmes, newspaper or magazine articles, or advice from a health professional were discussed. Assuming a model in which health promotion information is 'accepted' or 'rejected' on an individualistic basis omits recognition that such information is often disseminated within a social context and therefore is compared with other forms of knowledge and thus may be reformulated and adapted. Rather than necessarily prompting alteration in consumption patterns, an important aspect of discussion with friends and relatives seemed to be reassurance. The adage of 'If you did everything they said, you wouldn't eat anything' served to alleviate anxiety and reinforce the identity of 'us' possessing practical, common-sense knowledge with often limited possibilities for change, against 'them' trying to impose abstract and irrelevant knowledge.

Discussion

Participants in this study utilised a range of information sources, with those based on personal experience being the most highly valued. Participants' embodied knowledge, which was linked to their personal histories and experience of health and illness, formed the basis of their concepts of the relationship between food and health. While individuality was key to the discourses of embodied knowledge, association with class, gender and age positions was evident.

Although many in the study were following some aspects of healthy eating advice, few credited general advice as their source of inspiration. Participants reported that they found out through their own experience which consumption patterns suited them and they adapted their consumption to suit their own requirements as they felt necessary. Generally short-term priorities predominated.

The reliance on personal experience was compounded by distrust of official information sources. The abstract, generalisable body which forms the basis of health promotion discourse was rejected because participants felt it was not relevant to their own experience of 'my body'.

CONCLUSION

Consideration of the wider issues concerning healthy eating helps to contextualise ethnographic data. Contemporary concerns, such as the health effects of food processing, which do not fit in with the official line that healthy eating is a matter of individual choice, should not be dismissed by policy-makers or theorists as simply excuses for not following healthy eating advice. Such concerns have to be seen in the context of policies which have emphasised commercial freedom rather than commercial responsibility. For participants in this study, reliance on oneself and informal sources of knowledge offered some measure of control in the context of an information system that they perceived to be based on the needs of the producer rather than the consumer. Furthermore, issues such as the role of genetic susceptibility in illness should be more clearly discussed in health promotion material if it is to be taken seriously by the public, who have a knowledge which contradicts health promotion representations of aetiology.

The results from this study suggest that healthy eating advice is indeed rather hard to swallow and that people do not feel they are getting the information that they deserve.

NOTES

1 This chapter is based on data collected as part of the 'Concepts of Healthy Eating' (Lewisham) project, which was part of the Economic and Social Research Council's 'The Nation's Diet: The Social Science of Food Choice' research programme. The project was directed by Professor Pat Caplan, the field-work was conducted by Anne Keane and Anna Willetts (research associates).

2 Griggs (1986) comments that the milling industry lobbied the government to keep the extraction rate of flour low because high profits were made by selling extracted wheatgerm to patent medicine companies and bran for animal feed.

3 The Ministry of Food was set up at the start of the Second World War. It was amalgamated with the Ministry of Agriculture and Fisheries in 1955. Many have since argued that these should be separated in the interests of consumers.

4 For example the Coronary Prevention Group was set up in 1979. The London Food Commission (now called the Food Commission) was set up in 1985. The National Food Alliance was formed in 1985 to act as an umbrella organisation for a number of campaigning and professional groups concerned with food policy.

5 The Department of Health (1992) defines a Body Mass Index between 25 and 30 as 'overweight' and over 30 as 'obese'.

6 This comment refers to the original BSE controversy in 1989.

7 This point refers to general healthy eating advice. Risks to health which are perceived as immediate, such as salmonella infection in eggs, have much more dramatic effects on consumption patterns than on-going advice aimed at the prevention of chronic illness (Davison 1989, Miller and Reilly 1994b).

REFERENCES

Backett, K. (1992) 'Taboos and excesses: lay health moralities in middle-class families', *Sociology of Health & Illness* 14, 2: 255–74.

Cannon, G. (1987) *The Politics of Food*, London: Century Hutchinson Ltd.

Cannon, G. (1992) *Food and Health: The Experts Agree. An Analysis of One Hundred Authoritative Scientific Reports on Food, Nutrition and Public Health Published Throughout the World in Thirty Years, between 1961 and 1991*, London: Consumers' Association Ltd.

Cole-Hamilton, I. and Lang, T. (1986) *Tightening Belts – A Report on the Impact of Poverty on Food*, London: The London Food Commission.

Davison, C., Frankel, S. and Smith, G.D. (1992) 'The limits of lifestyle: re-assessing "fatalism" in the popular culture of illness prevention', *Social Science and Medicine* 34: 675–85.

Davison, C., Smith, G.D. and Frankel, S. (1991) 'Lay epidemiology and the prevention paradox: the implications of coronary candidacy for health education', *Sociology of Health & Illness*, 13, 1: 1–19.

Department of Health (1992) *The Health of the Nation: A Strategy for Health in England*, London: HMSO.

—— (1995) *Fit for the Future: Second Progress Report on the Health of the Nation*, London: Department of Health.

—— (1996) *Eat Well II: A Progress Report from the Nutrition Task Force on the Action Plan to Achieve the Health of the Nation Targets on Diet and Nutrition*, London: Department of Health.

Dibb, S. (1992) 'Slimming scandal', *The Food Magazine* February/April: 8–9.

Dobson, B., Beardsworth, A., Keil, T. and Walker, R. (1994) *Diet, Choice and Poverty: Social, Cultural and Nutritional Aspects of Food Consumption among Low-income Families*, London: Family Policy Studies Centre.

Farrant, W. and Russell, J. (1986) *The Politics of Health Information: 'Beating Heart Disease' as a Case Study of Health Education Publications*, London: Institute of Education.

Fine, B. and Wright, J. (1991) *Digesting the Food and Information Systems*, Discussion Papers in Economics 7/91, London: Department of Economics, Birkbeck College, University of London.

The Food Commission (1994) 'Selling food to kids', *Living Earth and the Food Magazine* Oct.: 14–15.

Garner, D. and Wooley, S. (1991) 'Confronting the failure of behavioral and dietary treatments for obesity', *Clinical Psychology Review* 11: 729–80.

Griggs, B. (1986) *The Food Factor: An Account of the Nutrition Revolution*, London: Penguin Books.

Leather, S. (1992) 'Less money, less choice: poverty and diet in the UK today', pp. 72–94 in National Consumer Council (ed.), *Your Food: Whose Choice?* London: HMSO.

Lobstein, T. (1990) 'The corporate clinic', *The Food Magazine* Oct./Dec.: 22–3.

—— (1991) *The Nutrition of Women on Low Incomes*, London: The Food Commission.

Longfield, J. (1992) 'Advertising and labelling: how much influence?' pp. 49–71 in National Consumer Council (ed.) *Your Food: Whose Choice?* London: HMSO.

Lupton, D. (1995) *The Imperative of Health: Public Health and the Regulated Body*, London: Sage.

Lupton, D. and Chapman, S. (1995) '"A healthy lifestyle might be the death of you": discourses on diet, cholesterol control and heart disease among the lay public', *Sociology of Health and Illness* 14, 4: 477–94.

Miller, D. and Reilly, J. (1994a) *Food 'Scares' in the Media*, Glasgow University: The Glasgow University Media Group in association with the MRC Medical Sociology Unit.

—— (1994b) *The Role of the Media in the Emergence of Food Panics*, Report for 'The Nation's Diet' Research Programme, Department of Sociology, University of Glasgow.

Mills, M. (1992) *The Politics of Dietary Change*, Aldershot: Dartmouth Publishing Co. Ltd.

National Children's Home (1991) *NCH Poverty and Nutrition Survey*, London: National Children's Home.

National Food Alliance (1995) *Nutrition Task Force: Goodbye or Good Riddance?*, Update No. 16: 1.

Smith, M.J. (1991), 'From policy community to issue network: salmonella in eggs and the new politics of food', *Public Administration*, 69: 235–55.

West, R. (1994) *Obesity*, London: Office of Health Economics.

Williams, S. (1995) 'Theorising class, health and lifestyles: can Bourdieu help us?' *Sociology of Health and Illness* 17, 5: 577–604.

Wilson, G. (1989) 'Family food systems, preventative health and dietary change: a policy to increase the health divide', *Journal of Social Policy* 18: 167–85.

Chapter 10

Being told what to eat

Conversations in a Diabetes Day Centre

Simon Cohn

Recently it has been recognised that an anthropological concern with food would benefit from alliance with the renewed interest in the phenomenological concepts of embodiment and lived experience (Lupton 1996). Previous work that tended to focus on the interpretation of the symbolic values of food and meals echoed the general trend of utilising cultural events and habits as texts to be read. This domination of symbolic approaches has proved very powerful, providing classic studies that have revealed some of the cultural rules that underlie what were assumed to be merely nutritional requirements (Lévi-Strauss 1965 and Douglas 1972 being the obvious examples). However, in the process of unravelling and revealing cultural patterns this perspective has served to remove the actor from view; by concentrating on the textual aspects of food culture, individual dietary choices, the experience of eating and how these relate to personal ideas about the self and the body are ignored.

The current influence of Heidegger and psychoanalytic theory in the social sciences can be seen as complementary to post-structuralists' generally singular concern with textuality through the stress on the individual in the lived world. Although Heidegger adopts a somewhat metaphysical claim for an existentially authentic self, the appeal of this perspective is a combined recognition of social influence and that the individual is potentially a free agent. It is thereby a rejection of the western philosophical premise of an a priori self divorced from experience and hence sympathetic to social constructionist approaches. However, in contrast to a Foucauldian depiction of the body as the supreme site of pervasive power, a stress on existence as experience places the self as part of the world – and denies any abstraction from it (Csordas 1994).

Arguably the true challenge is not simply a recognition of the impossibility of dividing the body from the self, or the self from the social, but that humans are, through technologies of symbolism, reflexive. This, then, enables individuals to project a sense of themselves, of the world and, crucially, their own place in it.

This chapter aims to address the concepts of embodied experience and food choice through one example of a patient talking with both a medical professional and myself. Rather than claiming that biomedical values are inscribed upon the body, thus rendering the individual passive, the discussion suggests ways in which meanings are interpreted and lived out. What it illustrates is how an apparently dominant 'cultural script', here in the form of biomedical instruction about what to eat and ultimately how to live, is transcribed, experienced and acted through. The context is the link between food and health, or rather, food and illness, and the case is one of a diabetic.[1]

A CONCEPT OF BALANCE

Health and the body are inevitably concepts dominated by moral criteria. They are both uniquely individual concerns that are also governed by a vast scope of social judgement. Historically, biomedicine has tended to neglect a link between the body and the social. Its application is an endeavour for optimal order and physiological control which has led to the suppression of individuality and hence the division of the disease from the person.[2] Thus, individuals are transmuted into cases, and bodies divided into their constituent parts. However, the growing discourse on 'the duty to be healthy' initiated by recent health education policies (Bunton and Macdonald 1992), contextualised within broader ecological models of causes and treatments of many conditions (Ashton and Seymour 1988), has led to a call for more personal responsibility. Health now calls for effort and discipline, and is presented as a means for self-realisation and salvation, placing the individual not only under the gaze of biomedicine, but also within its moral framework.

Diabetes, which takes two main forms, is, in essence, a metabolic condition in which the basic building block of carbohydrates, sugar, is absorbed into the bloodstream but not successfully utilised. The resulting wayward levels can in the short term lead to acute illness, and in the long term lead to serious complications.

Prolonged high blood sugar levels damage nerve tissue and blood vessels, which can cause blindness and give rise to the need for foot amputation. Insulin secreted in the pancreas, which acts on the blood sugar, is either not produced or not produced sufficiently.

Biomedical treatment is an attempt artificially to recreate the metabolic balance between food intake and its utilisation, and may or may not include the administering of animal or synthetic insulin by injection. In all cases food intake needs constantly to be under check, ensuring that foods high in refined sugars are eliminated as far as possible, that body weight is kept stable around average on the body-mass index and that an overall equilibrium is achieved between food intake, metabolic process and any medication taken. The key to this conception is that internal homeostatic processes are faulty, and that their mimicry can only be achieved by external influence. For diabetes, the biomedical objective is the maintenance of normal blood sugar levels through a life-embracing regimen. Since the condition is chronic the regimen is perpetual. Diet, medication and exercise are all to be objectified through self-regulation and self-surveillance. The difficulty with such a conception for patients is that the internal body, which usually is not part of people's sense of self, is brought to the fore, and made both visible and dominant. Thus, the internal body and the self as it is experienced in the world are forced into confrontation through the application of an assessment of balance. This is indeed, as Hahn (1985) has described, medicine of an internal world.

Studies of many differing non-biomedical belief systems illustrate links between ideas concerning food with general concepts of health. The over-riding motif tends to be one of balance, in which food is regarded as part of a set of elements that can influence internal humoral equilibrium. While humoral theories vary in the number of dimensions that are incorporated, for example in Latin America equilibrium is conceived between four opposing forces (Foster 1987) and in China between five (Anderson 1988), most can be reduced to a basic antagonism between categories of 'hot' and 'cold' (Mennell *et al.* 1992: 43). The West had its own version in the form of the Hippocratic Theory (Helman 1992: 18), dominant prior to the rise of biomedicine, in which four bodily substances, blood, phlegm, yellow bile and black bile, were associated with opposing elemental forces.

Humoral models provide a conception of the body in which the internal state of the self is directly related to the external social world; they are essentially moral representations. What is of interest is how humoral characteristics are not restricted to one arena, but are evaluations made over a broad scope seen to influence health. Since, by implication, sickness is defined as being out of balance, a physical or mental abnormality is regarded as a symptom of disequilibrium. In such cases as illness food is often presented as a chief mechanism for readjustment. While the cause of an illness may be externally assigned, for example to witchcraft or the spirits, a humoral model privileges individual control through the ability to determine appropriate corrective foodstuffs. By claiming the holistic integration of many diverse factors one arena can be compensated for by another: the social world and the individual as free agent are thereby united. Although certain factors may be regarded as beyond control, individual acts such as food choice allow for personal agency. Such models provide the promise of control with food placed as one such technique for regaining stasis and asserting authority in the world.

Although the biomedical conception of diabetes, along with a range of other lifestyle conditions, includes a holistic model, and although this now stresses the dimension of individual agency under the label of self-care, crucially it lacks the moral map shared by patient and healer that is the basis of these humoral models.

Values placed upon sugar play an important part in the disjunction between the biomedical and lay models that arise during the treatment of diabetes. Fischler (1987) has suggested that the universal fondness for sweet foods can be attributed to a biologically based 'nutritional wisdom' that underlies cultural models of balance. However, his suggestion of an adaptive environmental strategy provides little more than a functional component of broader and more complex influences on cultural habits. Mintz (1985), in charting the history of refined sugar in England, has shown how sugar has shifted from a status of high value to being conceived of as a common and essential component of diet amongst the working classes. In so doing he demonstrates how the 'taste' for a food item is as much determined by its symbolic value as availability or an innate preference.

This reclassification of sugar has continued in the West, however, not merely from preciousness to profane, but towards one of imminent danger. Combined with other food types, the over-consumption of sugar is now equated with a range of medical conditions.[3] The following discussion relates to this shifting of the status of food by showing how sweet foods are differently conceived of by patients and biomedicine. Many patients continue to perceive sugar as central to their diet symbolising both pleasure and necessity. Sugar is seen to be an important component in maintaining balance within a humoral model based on an underlying theme of labour and consumption and a body-as-machine model that this implies. The medical profession, however, now regards the excessive intake of refined sugars as dangerous. Diabetes is conceived of as a lifestyle disease in which an inappropriate diet severely threatens the natural balance between an internal metabolism and the outside world.

BEING TOLD: ADVICE AND INSTRUCTION

In the context of the biomedical management of diabetes, balance is not restricted to the components of a meal, or the general assessment of food categories over time, but includes the relationship between food and other aspects of lifestyle. Specifically, treatment usually consists of a combination of medication, either tablets or insulin, with diet and exercise. Since diabetes is the failure of the body to convert blood sugars into other forms for use and storage, the combined regimen is designed to reduce blood sugar levels by other means. As a script it appears to provide the opportunity for individual autonomy and control.

Given that diabetes, like many other conditions, is now conceived to be a condition that can only be addressed through self-care, the emphasis has shifted from delivering instructions to giving advice. Advice is imparted as a gift during education sessions in the hope that patients will see their own way to health. Although patients may be given general advice about how they should live, such as to take regular exercise, health professionals make a point of saying that patients are advised about their diet. While this action is located within the current philosophy of empowerment it effectively denies reciprocity in dialogue, and instead transfers not only information but also obligation. To advise in this way is effectively to issue instruction, even though it uses a more amiable vocabulary. Thus, to advise also communicates from the biomedical perspective a moral attribute to the state of the body and the circumstances of the self in the world.

Many diabetic patients tend not to respond to the broad treatment philosophy. Their expectations of treatment are solely those of intervention and medication, and they feel that other dimensions, such as diet and exercise, are merely part of a rather tiresome health promotion message. For this reason, health professionals repeatedly stress that 'diet is part of the treatment, indeed, it *is* the treatment' since it is a primary, and the most manipulable, means of controlling blood sugar. For patients, who tend to have restricted expectations of biomedical therapy, the promotion of a healthy, balanced and largely sugar-free diet falls outside the remit of medical expertise, and, while not dismissed, is not credited with the same degree of significance as insulin or tablets. Food is felt to remain within a personal and social domain, not a medical one. As many commentators report, the claim that this knowledge is scientific and privileged is repeatedly undermined by contradictory messages. Food is one such topic of reinterpretation, with patients ruefully commenting on food scares coupled with contradictory advertising campaigns. Thus, lifestyle advice, as opposed to the more technical medication, is seen as more legitimately open for review.

The rest of this paper will be based on excerpts from one of many tape-recordings made during two years of observation in a London hospital. It illustrates how a patient receives dietary advice, and how this is only partially integrated into a broader set of life-experiences. Margot is representative of many of the patients, not only because of her personal profile and history of diabetes, but in the ways she and the medical staff respond to each other. The exchange is at one level uneventful, proceeding without any serious misunderstandings or hostility. However, at another level the conversation reveals the subtle strategies employed by both nurse and patient in accommodating their beliefs and agendas within the structure of the interaction.

Margot and her diabetes

Margot, a 56-year-old woman born in Jamaica who came to London in 1962 with her husband, enters a room in the Diabetes Day Centre of a hospital. She wears a smart two-piece purple suit and a turquoise hat. Her experience is typical: diagnosed with Type II, known also as maturity-onset diabetes eleven years ago, she went to her doctor with a range of symptoms but not suspecting that combined they suggested the diagnosis. She was at first put on a weight-reducing diet, cutting out all foods that contain a lot of sugar and increasing those high in fibre, in the hope that this would control her blood sugar levels. This action did not prove adequate and she was rapidly put on to oral medications both to slow the absorption rate of food and to stimulate the production of insulin. This, combined with the diet, exercise and home-monitoring of blood glucose levels, was generally successful. However, after a number of years the symptoms of tiredness, thirst and skin inflammation returned, and it was decided that insulin needed to become part of the regimen. She has been injecting the insulin morning and evening for a little over a year now. Margot settles while the specialist nurse, responsible for the daily running of the Centre, reads through the notes. These nurses, three at the Centre, play a crucial role, bridging the gap between providing purely technical instruction, as the doctors do, and more general caring advice. The specialist nurses describe themselves as being 'up against the coal face', having to deal with the constant distress and difficulties of an ever-increasing number of patients.

Margot and the nurse say 'Hello' to each other and the nurse continues: 'I'll give you this first to look at', handing the patient a pamphlet on dietary advice for diabetics produced by one of the drug companies. She goes on: 'OK, just remind me again, the stick that you use to test your urine . . . ?'

'Pink ones . . . ', the patient replies, while handing over her home diary in which she records the results.

'So, no negatives at all . . . right . . . so one light . . . and the rest medium and dark. Not very good is it?' comments the nurse.

'No . . . ', the patient chuckles with embarrassment, and tries to offer an explanation: 'Some days, I test it and it came out pink and I says "Oh good". But by the end of the day it's gone. . . . I think sometimes it depends on how active I am, or how much I'm worrying about the bills or whatever. If I have a cold or a virus I'm told it does stay for quite some time . . . so whether that's still lurking in the body I don't know. I've given up', she pauses with hesitation, ' . . . bothering.'

'Bothering? About what in particular?' the nurse asks with some alarm, obviously worried that the patient might be slackening the regimen.

'Well, I've got to inject myself morning and night and if I'm trying to do the right things and it's not getting any better I don't want to worry myself for ages . . . '

'Umm . . . the thing is to look and find out why this is happening, really.' The nurse hopes to encourage self-care, but recognises that it can lead to extreme anxiety.

'It's a bit disconcerting at times . . . trying to stick to the diet', the patient interjects.

'Mmm?'

'I mean, nothing is happening . . . '

'Right, OK. What about your weight?'

'It fluctuates. . . . One week. Then another . . . sometimes it's stable. . . . I don't think I'll ever get to the weight you want . . . ', admits the patient in a meek tone.

'Can I check your blood sugar today? What time did you have breakfast?' asks the nurse, wanting to know in case it affects the reading. She gets things ready: the small glucose meter, the sensitive strips for a drop of the patient's blood and a box of tissues.

'About nine', the patient replies while holding out a finger to be pricked.

'And what did you have?' A small drop of blood is swiftly extracted and placed onto a tiny strip inserted into a credit-card sized electronic meter.

'Boiled egg and two slices of toast.'

'Do you get hungry at this time in the morning?' asks the nurse, contemplating whether the insulin doses are causing excessive lowering of glucose levels.

'Umm', nods the patient. The machine beeps, announcing that a successful reading has been made. The nurse glances over and says, 'It isn't good. 17.9.'[4]

'Uhh!!'

'The thing is we could increase the insulin to help the blood sugar but that will in turn make you put on more weight, which just makes the problem worse. Do you feel tired at the moment? Thirsty?'

'I can usually tell when the sugar is up because of tiredness . . . '

The nurse reviews the notes once again and asks 'Were you on insulin from the beginning?'

'No, I was first on tablets, as many as six a day and they just told me. . . . You see I was at work at the time and I think my job was very stressful. . . . I didn't really want to go on insulin but the doctor said to me "Mrs T, we're recommending you to go on insulin. . . . There's the reading. . . . Either you take the insulin or you take the consequences. . . . " I . . . I . . . just couldn't handle it. . . . I asked for a month to think about it, and it wasn't getting any better and eventually it stabilised it. . . . My mom was very ill at home, there was a lot of things worrying me and I had a lot to cope with and it just crept up and up.'

Severity is often measured by many patients in terms of the number of tablets or frequency of insulin injections. In fact, since the diabetic regimen is designed to imitate a dynamic process, the number of tablets or injections has increased with technical developments, in order to supply a more continuous quantity of medication.

This opening section of the exchange is typical. The nurse's questions and comments revolve around the state of the diabetes, which, although conceived of as an all-encompassing disease, is objectified as a number to be read, a thing to be scrutinised. The nurse aims to establish the current state of the diabetes so that appropriate and relevant advice can be matched to it. The patient replies dutifully enough to the questions, but at every opportunity discusses the predicament of herself in the world, her worries and her stresses, with references to her diabetic condition only made as part of these.

MEASURING THE PLEASURE OF FOOD

Dietary advice for people with diabetes has changed over recent years. Old regimen instructions demanded that all foodstuffs were weighed and their energy content calculated according to standard tables. Everything was assigned a specific value, and patients were expected physically to weigh each constituent of every meal (see, for example, Lawrence 1965). This fashion of numerical quantification has now been relaxed with the realisation that it is impossible to quantify every factor in what is now conceived of as a lifestyle disease, and that, far from assisting patients, the strategy was itself a major cause of distress that impeded compliance. The focus now is on education, integrating medical advice within the patient's existing lifestyle rather than attempting to supplant it.

The nurse specialist decides to review Margot's diet in detail to see if any further advice need be given. 'Can you just take me through a general day, what you would have to eat . . . ?'

'It depends on what time I get up really. Normally I'll have cereal, and one or two slices of toast . . . '

'Right. . . . So what cereal do you have?'

'Bran Flakes . . . a bowl.'

'How big is a bowl?'

'Smallish bowl, might just . . . put it this way, about three ounces . . . because it's light.'

'So a cereal bowl . . . Is it piled up or level to the top?'

'Sometimes level, sometimes not . . . '

'And you have toast with that as well? How many slices?'

'Two.'

'Two. . . . Is that brown bread? Right. What about lunch?'

What appears as pedantic and trivial questioning serves three main functions. It provides a listing of foods so that any unsuitable components might be detected. It also re-introduces the diet to the patient, objectifying it out of experience as susceptible to, and valid for, medical scrutiny. Finally, the run-through offers insight into a patient's routines of living and general lifestyle; the diet is seen to provide a patient profile upon which to act.

'I find I don't always have lunch. . . . I tend to have a cup of tea or something, crackers or a sandwich, and then I'll have the main meal in the evening. . . . Sometimes some cheese . . . '

'Right, and what type of things do you have for your evening meal?' prompts the nurse.

'Again it varies, it could be fish, chicken, sometimes I cook . . . umm, sometimes those soya bean chunks from the health shop. . . . Something with root vegetables', the patient replies, hoping to gain approval by listing foods regularly suggested by the Centre.

'And how do you cook the fish?'

'Mainly steam it in a bit of foil, normally with marge or whatever, sometimes I'll use olive oil.'

'Right . . . ' the nurse replies somewhat sceptically, the response being unnaturally near to ideal.

' . . . then I'll have my mixture of vegetables: carrots, cabbage . . . it all just depends, not every day the same thing . . . ' continues the patient with a faultless list of recommended foods.

'Do you have potatoes with it?'

'Well . . . sometimes rice. Strange that I don't seem to eat as much as I used to. Put it this way, when the family was around you cook a lot, but now I don't bother, I'd rather cook potatoes or green bananas, you know, from the West Indian shop, than cook rice . . . '

'Umm, right. Do you tend to eat a lot of cheese?' the nurse asks, nothing that could become subject for castigation having been revealed.

'I wouldn't say I eat a lot . . . just if it's in the house and I feel like it. . . . But I eat a lot of nuts.' It is likely that the patient here presumes that nuts, associated with health food shops and 'natural' products, will give further proof that she is complying with the diet.

'Nuts?' the specialist nurse presses with an air of disbelief, immediately communicating that an error has been made.

'Yes', comes a hesitant reply.

'Right, what type of nuts?' The nurse has found an undesirable item, and will now make use of it.

'Varies from cashew nuts to peanuts', answers the patient, aware that, whether truthful or merely included to gain approval, a confession will have to be made.

'Right, because those are very high in fat and they're very high in calories. . . . Do you know what one single peanut is in calories?'

'No.'

'It's six calories.'

'One little nut?'

'One nut. They're wicked they are.'

'Oh, I won't say any more. That's my weakness . . . '

The current biomedical advice for people with diabetes is to 'eat sensibly, eat healthily'. The stringent nature of previous dietary instruction is further sweetened by an agreement that 'a treat once in a while does no harm'. It is in this context that the patient continues:

'Sometimes I have some cake, but only a small slice . . . '

'Well, how small?' enquires the nurse with some scepticism.

'Oh, could be as thin as that' answers the patient, with her thumb and first finger just a couple of centimetres apart. 'Isn't that small?'

'Right. A treat once in a while is fine.'

Such an absolution as this is interpreted by patients as a recognition of their own philosophy. What health professionals denote is that since the objective is to 'live a normal life' patients should not become over-obsessed and not be excluded from special occasion foods such as at weddings and birthdays. A treat for patients, however, is often the regular, habitual tonic that they use as a focus in their day-to-day lives. It is tempting to think that for diabetics it is because certain foods should be eliminated that they are desired. However, many state that sweet foods, such as confectioneries and cakes, were regarded as personal rewards even prior to diagnosis. These special foods are defined not solely by their sweetness, but in combination with their place in people's diets as extras: not satisfying hunger so much as providing sensual pleasure at certain times in daily routines. This reward dimension is fully incorporated into the rhythms of their lives, supplying markers between periods of labour, such as mid-morning breaks or afternoon snacks. That it is precisely these which are banned is interpreted as belief-affirming; treats always were seen as transgressions from labour, and the medical advice derived from the diabetes merely confirms their status. When pressed, patients admit that they are aware the advice does not really condone regular misdeeds. Yet, leaving the message sufficiently unquestioned serves to absolve them morally. Margot, in the above exchange, doesn't actually state how many times she has a small slice of cake. And the nurse, likewise, does not press further. The advice is given, the patient signals that she knows what the advice is, and the business of whether she actually lives by it is left ambiguous. Remaining unexamined, the issue of what constitutes a treat can continue as part of a gentle delusion. This is, then, a strategy to integrate the advice within patients' lifestyle rather than dictating advice that directly brings about lifestyle modifications.

This exchange between patient and professional illustrates how food is focused on as the means of achieving control and a direct way of regulating physiology. Dietary advice is presented positively – as a means of regaining balance and harmony. In practice, the majority of patients fail to keep within the desired range of blood sugar levels, and although medication can easily be altered, it is the diet that is the first thing to come under scrutiny. In this way food, the means of success, rapidly comes to serve also as a means of symbolising guilt and failure. Its dual function is useful in this way to both professional and patient, since it provides a common site on which both can focus, distilling the vast range of possible lifestyle factors into clear elements that can be acted upon. From the biomedical perspective food is part of a biochemical-ecological model of the body that links not only the outside with the inside, but also the free will of the person with the state of the body. For the patient, food provides a subject matter to demonstrate compliance and gain approval, and also a detached topic upon which medical disdain can be accommodated. It is the fact that food lies on this interface which makes it so potentially dangerous.

THE BODY TALKING

Having had her appointment with the nurse specialist, I ask Margot if she would mind just a few minutes for a further chat with me. I explain that I'm doing some research, that I'll continue to tape-record if that's OK, but that I was keen to hear her views without any of the staff present. She readily agrees, as do most patients.

> After the brief introduction, I ask, ' . . . and I was just wondering if you feel in control of it all, or not?'
>
> 'I don't think so. I don't think so because when I talk to some people who are and I say "I eat so and so, or do so and so" they say "but you shouldn't, because I don't" and that makes me feel, well, it's you who are not taking care of the diabetes, that is why it goes up all the time and isn't stabilising. . . . You know?'

It is curious, but typical, how Margot shifts from using the first to using the second person. It is as though the first person is reserved for actions and experiences, thereby demanding statements about her body to be constructed differently, achieving a detachment between the self and body. She goes on:

> 'I'll get up in the morning and I will forget to take the insulin, maybe until I'm eating, so I'm not in control. If I was in control I would know I get out of bed, I have my bath, I take my insulin then breakfast, but sometimes I start eating and I remember that I haven't done it, and then I've got to rush upstairs. . . . So I wouldn't say that I am in control.'
>
> 'But it doesn't sound as though diabetes rules your life either; you're not obsessed?' I enquire.

'No, I'm not, and probably that in itself might be dangerous.
... It's like eating a cake. Some people wouldn't touch anything
sweet because they know they shouldn't. . . . Now, I think, what
the heck, a little bit won't hurt, you know, and I take it.'

There is trust in this statement. Margot had insisted to the nurse
that she only ate very small quantities of cake, yet here implies that
its consumption is a regular occurrence.

I respond without any surprise or criticism, but nevertheless try
and press the issue a little further: 'Do you really think a little
bit won't hurt or are you just trying to convince yourself?'
'I think I do it to convince myself, because I know. . . . I feel
the body needs a certain amount of sugar. . . . I don't take sugar
in my tea, I eat a lot of carrots, I eat things that will produce
certain amounts of sugar, but because sometimes I get so tired
I think, well, the energy isn't there, the body's trying to tell me
something. So if I eat a bit of cake or if I have a couple of sweet
biscuits or whatever, it balances it out.'

Sugar is in this instance seen to provide energy. Lethargy, which
may actually be a result of not being able to utilise high levels
of blood sugar, is interpreted as an indication that sustenance
is needed. The body requires sugar, tells Margot, and she obliges.
In this context, sugar, as well as being a treat, is also seen as a
necessity. The emotional and psychological satisfaction of a
reward ritual is allied with a belief that it also serves a bodily
demand. The humoral characteristics of this belief-system, that
sugar supplies both comfort and energy, is combined in the notion
that sweet foods offer replenishment. In Margot's model, sugar
as a tonic and as a top-up are one and the same thing. Underlying
this is the idea of utilisation; the pleasure of a sweet food is the
re-establishment of potential. This model is seen to compete with
the biomedical advice:

'You see the experts are saying this is what you must do and my
mind is saying otherwise. . . . So, who is true I don't know. . . .
They must know what they're talking about but I don't feel . . .
that I could really conform . . . '. I sense some relief in her
consistent use of 'they' thereby confirming that however she
categorises me, she does not see me as part of the medical
expertise. I chuckle a response, colluding as I do with this
division between Us and Them, and continue: 'Well, do you

think of yourself as healthy although you've got diabetes? Or do you see yourself as ill?'

'Err . . . sometimes I do . . . because I feel tired. Then I start getting the headaches . . . but what I do to overcome that. . . . I make sure I get regular check-ups. . . . If for any reason I feel any aches and pains I go to my doctor, but I feel well, I'm healthy. . . . It's just these dumb blood sugars will not settle itself. . . . But I don't play on it. Some people say "I'm diabetic and I can't do this and I can't do that." I don't think of it that way. . . . It is a condition that I've got to try and live with . . . and I'm not going to let that stop me from doing certain things. That's how I look at it.'

'Do you resent the fact that the nurses and doctors say it's up to you . . . ?'

'No, no, because it's my body and they can only advise me what to do, and it's up to me to do it or not . . . so if it goes against me and anything happens I blame myself.' It occurs to me that, unfortunately, so often the power of self-care philosophy is only experienced in the negative.

'Has anyone told you of any effects it might mean?' I urge.

'Yes, I know all that. I know because my sister, she's diabetic, and she's going to have a cataract removed and some people develop all sorts of things. I know I have arthritis but I developed that before I had diabetes so I wouldn't put that down and say "because I'm diabetic I've got that . . . " you know?'

I recall some of the in-patients suffering from gangrene that follows nerve and blood vessel damage while Margot continues: 'I cannot honestly say my eyes have deteriorated as a result', and I'm relieved that her images are not the same as mine.

'Do you think getting those complications is not simply due to blood sugars?' I ask.

'That aspect of it I put down to my Christian beliefs. . . . I believe that you get what you pray for. . . . I ask God to sustain me, to give me the strength to live with diabetes . . . '

'But do you always get what you pray for?' I press.

'Not always. I take your point, but I believe God gives you what He thinks is best for you . . . and if what you pray for is in tune with His will, it happens.'

Margot does not hold her beliefs as in conflict with the messages she gets from the health professionals. Rather, the advice that she is given is experienced as providing a touchstone specific to her ideas of the body with diabetes. Although from the biomedical perspective it is a lifestyle disease, for Margot and many other patients, it is merely a breakdown of one context of the body, that requires a particular kind of replenishment. And Margot is confident that the body, her body, has a way of telling her what it needs.

DISEASED SELF AS OTHER

Given that diabetes and the body are not necessarily central to people's sense of self as it is lived, their attribution often illustrates ways in which the internal disease is placed within the world as it is experienced. Hence, in reply to my question asking what she thinks caused the diabetes, Margot states at length:

'I'm convinced it was a state of depression. I had broken up with a friend and it was very painful, and I had a glimpse of what a recluse could be like, because I didn't want to trust anybody, me, I didn't want to talk to anybody, I just wanted to go to work and come back. . . . I tell you, I must have been like this for months and one night I went to bed and I felt as though I wanted to be sick. I got up and went to the bathroom and having gone there, I don't know for how long I was in there, I got up from the bathroom floor. Then, about six months later, I was talking to my sister about how I was feeling and there was a lady in the front of the bus, she says, "Excuse me, if you think I'm a bit rude, but from what I hear you should go and see your GP."

'I went and tested it and it was 20. And that's how I know that mine was brought on because of the depressive state I was in. . . . Because I'm not really one of those people who go on moaning and that. . . . I try to fight things and keep above them . . . but that really hit me hard. I started really shaking it off last year. You can't trust people, that's why anything I have to say now I just say to myself or to above . . . you just can't trust . . . you see I don't have many friends. . . . I talk to everybody but I would never trust anyone enough to tell them anything secret of mine, never ever again.'

For Margot, the diabetes is a physical expression of her social collapse. This synchronicity between body and self is derived from an underlying need of replenishment. Sadness and depression felt by Margot is equivalent to the body lacking energy. Margot expresses the view that her problem is not diabetes but her over-riding sense of loneliness and feeling betrayed. It is this betrayal that caused the depression and her physical condition, and it is this betrayal that she hopes she is getting over.

> 'I'm getting these things out of my system . . . and now I couldn't give two hoots. . . . That's the long and short of how I feel my diabetes has developed. . . . And a strange thing is that I was speaking to [the nurse] and I said to her "Now and again I buy West Indian food which is very starchy", and I asked her if she thinks that is why I have it, and she said: "No it's hereditary". . . . Well, I don't know if that's true or not, but she's the expert, so I just have to take her words for it. . . . But once you have diabetes, this is where I'm convinced about the diet, once you have it you have to be careful about what you eat. . . . And don't tell anyone, but I still have a chocolate bar every day.'

Given that food is placed between what patients see as medical provision and an important component of their life beyond medical encounters it becomes increasingly difficult to maintain any distinction between the diseased and the true self. Keeping to the lifestyle advice is to satisfy the medical profession and to acknowledge an enduring sick identity. This generally passive response is countered by a strong desire not to be a permanently ill person. Spurning dietary advice can be a form of resistance not so much to biomedical authority but to a recognition of the self as diseased. Having a treat, the chocolate, some cake, is a recognition and an affirmation of the self as it always has been, a self not betrayed by others, with the usual routines, usual requirements and usual balance.

CONCLUSION

The experience that lifestyle advice serves to divide the self that has diabetes from the self that wishes to remain as it was is at odds with the biomedical philosophy contending that a sense of internalisation provides the solution: taking the medication, controlling the intake of food and having regular exercise all being seen as demonstrable ways of integrating the disease within a concept of personhood. Patients such as Margot do not experience this promise of independence, since their very acts of freedom are being surveyed. The paradox is that food is offered by biomedicine as a primary forum for control yet for patients is regarded as a key provision of self-expression and self-comfort.

This illustration raises a number of key issues. Discussions over embodiment have claimed that it is through the body and its praxis that a sense of self is often derived. The study of people who are chronically ill, however, demonstrates how an affected body can be divorced from a notion of the self. It is not that the body is denied, or that it is split apart by some Cartesian dualism, but that it can itself embody disorder, fragmentation or disequilibrium. Thus, for Margot the diabetes is her life's distresses made physical, and the body is thereby made alien. As such, the condition is tangible, and though not necessarily controlled in the biomedical sense, is made acceptable to Margot.

The use of this one case has shown also how the concepts of disease and the body, and the role of food, are differently perceived by health care professionals and patients. Within the current biomedical model of disease food has increasingly become central in linking lifestyle with physiology. It is seen to provide both reasons for imbalance and disease, and also a mechanism for its readjustment. Dietary advice is given in order that the person and the disease are integrated and individually controlled.

For patients, ideas of food and health remain based on concepts of potential, energy and replenishment. The exchange between Margot and myself revealed how ideas of the illness were related to a concept of the self as experienced in activity beyond the Diabetes Day Centre, establishing how, for patients, food and the body are part of a different explanatory model. Here there is a symbolic depth by which regulation and balance are not merely measurements accessible to science, but include assessments of a social and moral order. The result is not that patients ignore biomedical advice, or deliberately live contrary to it, but that they see this advice as corresponding specifically to the diseased body. This body is one that has already been divorced from their sense of self since it has absorbed and responded to disequilibrium in their lived world.

NOTES

1 Field-work was carried out in a South London Diabetes Day Centre between 1993–5 for a doctoral thesis, funded by an ESRC studentship. Over this period direct observations were made in all types of medical encounter, many being tape-recorded, and I interviewed patients both before and after their contact with the medical staff.
2 This tenet is central to the biomedical conception of diabetes mellitus, which is diagnosed on the basis of blood sugar levels above what is considered the normal range, currently as determined by the World Health Organisation (WHO 1980).
3 The main biomedical conditions that some have classed as a single disease are obesity, heart disease and diabetes mellitus. However, such other ailments as tooth decay have also been included under the biomedical premise that a single cause means that medicine is ultimately dealing with a single disease.
4 Figures given by glucose meters register the amount of glucose in millimoles per litre of blood. The range for somebody who does not have diabetes fluctuates between 3 and 7.5 mml. Anything more than 10 mml implies that the metabolic system is not functioning well, and itself often serves as a diagnosis and definition of diabetes mellitus.

REFERENCES

Anderson, E.N. (1988) *The Food of China*, New Haven: Yale University Press.
Ashton, J. and Seymour, H. (1988) *The New Public Health*, Milton Keynes: Open University Press.
Bunton, R. and Macdonald, G. (eds.) (1993) *Health Promotion: Disciplines and Diversity*, London and New York: Routledge.
Csordas, T.J. (ed.) (1994) *Embodiment and Experience: The Existential Ground of Culture and Self*, Cambridge: Cambridge University Press.
Douglas, M. (1972) 'Deciphering a meal', *Daedalus* 101, 1: 61–81.
Fischler, C. (1987) 'Attitudes towards sugar and sweetness in historical and social perspective', in J. Dobbing (ed.) *Sweetness*, Berlin: Springer.
Foster, G.M. (1987) 'On the origin of humoral medicine in Latin America', *Medical Anthropology Quarterly* 1: 355–93.
Hahn, R.A. (1985) 'A world of internal medicine: portrait of an internist', in R.A. Hahn and A.D. Gaines (eds) *Physicians of Western Medicine*, Dordrecht: D. Reidel Publishing Co.
Helman, C.G. (1992) *Culture, Health and Illness: An Introduction for Health Professionals*, Oxford: Butterworth-Heinemann.
Lawrence, R. (1965) *The Diabetic Life*, London, Churchill Ltd.
Lévi-Strauss, C. (1965) 'The culinary triangle', *Partisan Review* 33: 586–95.
Lupton, D. (1996) *Food, the Body and the Self*, London: Sage.

Mennell, S., Murcott, A. and van Otterloo, A.H. (1992) *The Sociology of Food: Eating, Diet and Culture*, London: Sage.

Mintz, S.W. (1985) *Sweetness and Power: The Place of Sugar in Modern History*, New York: Viking.

World Health Organisation (1980) *Expert Committee on Diabetes Mellitus, Second Report*, Geneva: World Health Organisation.

Chapter 11

Health, eating and heart attacks

Glaswegian Punjabi women's thinking about everyday food

Hannah Bradby

This chapter discusses the ways in which young British Asian women understand food and health to be related. In particular the focus is on how a synthesis is made between the understandings that are recognisably 'western' and those that are clearly related to the Ayurvedic tradition of the Indian subcontinent. Studies of understandings of health among the ethnic majority have described how medical orthodoxy and lay understandings of health cannot be clearly distinguished from one another (Davison *et al.* 1991). Individuals in a mass society hold opinions that are modified versions of those of the health agencies in wider society. Although traces of a system of beliefs about health that pre-date current medical orthodoxy can be found (Helman 1990), lay populations generally show a thorough grasp of orthodox understandings of health and illness causation (Backett *et al.* 1994).

The special interest of young women of Punjabi origin for the study of how lay people conceptualise health is that they have been exposed to the medical orthodoxy of 'healthy eating' and they also have access to the folk beliefs of their forebears from the Indian subcontinent. A qualitative study of how women use the resources available to them in thinking about food and health illustrates the processes that occur when orthodox health messages are integrated with alternative models for considering food and health.

METHODS

This chapter is based on a study in Glasgow with young women of Punjabi origin who were asked about foods they thought were good and bad for health. A sample of forty-seven women aged

20 to 30 with South Asian names was drawn at random from a possible 70 women of the appropriate age and ethnicity on a general practice list in the north of Glasgow. Of these, thirty-two women were interviewed twice and these interviews were tape-recorded and transcribed. Interviews were conducted in English by the author, with five conducted by a colleague in Punjabi or Urdu, with the author present to take notes and occasionally prompt the line of questioning. The same colleague helped translate the interview schedule into Punjabi and the Punjabi or Urdu transcripts into English. Interview material was complemented by an extended period of participant observation in the private and public forums of Punjabi life in Glasgow, the former involving considerable participation in the lives of four key informants, and the latter centring around one of the city's Sikh temples and one of the mosques where weekly women's meetings were held (for more details see Bradby 1996).

The interviewees and respondents reflected the population of South Asian origin in Glasgow, being Punjabi speakers who traced their origins to the east or west Punjab; the majority were Muslims with an important minority of Sikhs and fewer Hindus. They included both married and unmarried women. The majority were British born, but a third were born in the subcontinent and either arrived in Britain as children (at various ages from 2 months to 11 years) or as adult brides.

FOOD AND HEALTH

Women reported eating a large variety of foods, and tended to divide them into 'our' foods (Asian) and 'your sort of foods' (Scottish or British). Their daily food reflected their Punjabi origins, consisting of *chapatti* or *roti* (unleavened round bread cooked on a griddle), accompanied by dishes of meat, vegetables or pulses cooked in a liquid sauce of spices, onions, ginger, garlic and chillies, and known generically as *saalan*, *dahl* (mainly lentil), *subsee* (mainly vegetable) or *ghosht* (mainly meat). The Punjabi food was generally eaten as the main meal of the day, with non-Asian food such as pizza or fish and chips introduced for variety two or three times a week.

Women's accounts showed that health was a powerful reason for explaining the rationale behind daily food choice. There were two models by which the health value of foods was assessed: one derived from the authority of a western medical view of the world and one from the authority of South Asian elders. The first model is referred to as *reductionist* because it relies upon certain elements of foodstuffs to explain effects upon particular parts of the body and the second as *systemic* because health is considered in terms of the effect of the whole food on the whole body in a way that is contingent upon many other variables. These were not terms that women themselves used, but are designations for systems that were conceptually distinct in women's accounts. In what follows, the authority that is attributed by women to the two means of assessing the health of foods is considered, together with the ways in which the two models related to one another.

The first type of explanation of why foods were good for health, the reductionist view, stated that a food was good because of something it contained that was also good in an intrinsic way. The good effect of the food was often related to its effect on a specific part of the body. The second, systemic, view referred to the effect of the whole food on the body, often relating this to the type of weather prevailing or the stage of life which the consumer had reached, in deducing whether or not the effect of the food was 'good'. The first type of answer relied on a largely dichotomous classification in which foods were either good or bad. The second type of answer was more complex, dependent on context and time, so a particular food might be good in one time and place for a certain person, but this could change. Thus one food could have several roles through time, and women were likely to talk of the maintenance of a balance of health, while taking other factors into consideration.

REDUCTIONIST MODEL: 'GOOD' AND 'BAD' CONSTITUENTS

Foods that women reported as being categorically good for health included fresh fruit and vegetables, dairy products, cereals and pulses. The reasons why these foods were good were more difficult to ascertain. Some women could offer only a tautological response, stating that these foods were good because they were good for you. Otherwise the answer was given in terms of the goodness of the nutrients that these foods contained. For instance, vegetables were identified as containing vitamins; fish, cheese, fromage frais and lentils were said to contain protein, and jacket potatoes, salad and brown bread were said to be good because they are full of fibre. Eating a diet with enough of the 'good' foods was said to ensure that one received the required amount of the 'good' vitamins and minerals. Foods that were said to contain iron, calcium and vitamins were necessarily good, and the 'good' effect of the vitamins and minerals was often not explained any further. A woman explained why she liked her children to eat fruit:

> I mean fruit has got a lot of calcium and iron and things as well, and vitamins. I mainly like to give them because I want them to have more vitamins.

Despite the lack of knowledge about them, the presence of vitamins in a food was a powerful reason for considering a food to have a beneficial effect on health and was used to explain the value of foods ranging from Ribena to *roti-saalan*. Foods that were said not to contain vitamins, such as chips and waffles, were said to be bad on this basis alone.

The reductionist model of food and health also identified foods whose effect was to compromise health, and the prime offenders in this respect were said to be fat and sugar. The foods that were identified as containing a lot of sugar and fat or 'cholesterol' were collectively referred to as 'junk food' and included ready-made items such as chocolate, biscuits, cakes, sweets, crisps, as well as fried snacks such as burgers, *pakoras* (deep fried, battered nuggets of meat, fish or vegetable) and chips.

Sugar was identified mainly as a problem for children's teeth and the foods that contained it were fizzy drinks and sweets. The other problem with sweets, ice-cream and soft drinks was that they contained little else that was reported as 'good'. As one mother put it, they are just 'watery stuff with no goodness in them'. Sugar was mentioned as an accompaniment to and even accomplice of fat, the 'really bad' food stuff:

> *Question*: And what foods are bad for your health?
> *Answer*: Chocolate biscuits and cakes, sweets, fried foods, you know.
> *Question*: And why are they bad for your health?
> *Answer*: Because they just fill you up with sugar and grease and fat you know. Sugar and carbohydrates are not really good for you . . . bad for your teeth and . . . make you put on weight.

Although sugar was admitted as necessary in some small part in the diet by some women, fat was talked of as an intrinsically bad food. This 'badness' meant that reduced quantities of fat rendered a food beneficial to health, and reduced-calorie foods such as low-fat spreads were frequently mentioned as being good for health. Indeed the 'badness' that fat imparted to food led one woman to say that she thought that the only good food was fruit because of its lack of fat. She, like many other women, used the word 'cholesterol' as a synonym for fat.

> In my knowledge I think the best thing is fruit . . . that's the best thing there is about, everything else is fattening and, ooooh, it gives you nothing, innit, too much cholesterol, too much that . . .

Foods that contained fat, such as chips, or that were said to have a fattening effect, such as banana, were therefore classified as bad, and this in turn became grounds for assuming that they lacked vitamins. Thus 'contains vitamins' became a metaphor for 'good'; and 'bad', being the opposite of 'good', implied a lack of vitamins.

Fatty and therefore 'bad' foods came in three guises. First, there were foods to which lots of fat was added during preparation, such as curries and some rice dishes that require oil, *ghee* (clarified butter) or margarine. Second, there were foods which are cooked in oil, including anything fried such as chips, fish, fish fingers, *paratha* (unleavened bread cooked with oil on a griddle), *pakora*, beefburgers and waffles. Third was meat, which was unusual in being the only food identified as fat-containing that was also named by some non-vegetarians as food that could be good for health. However, it was only felt to be 'healthy' within limits, and if eaten every day would mean the intake of too much fat. Meat is particularly interesting in terms of the ways of thinking dealt with here, and is more fully discussed later.

The effects which fat was felt to have on the body, and which led to its vilification as a foodstuff, were its contribution to increased body weight and to 'heart trouble'. Fried foods, heavy foods, *ghee* and butter were all identified as 'bad' or 'dangerous' for the heart by promoting or even causing heart disease. Some felt that this 'bad' effect was brought about through 'cholesterol', although what 'cholesterol' was beyond being 'bad fat' was not made clear. It was suggested that vegetable oil had less fat and/or less cholesterol compared with butter or *ghee* and therefore represented a healthier option. The reductionist model did not offer an understanding of the causation of heart attacks. Nonetheless most respondents said that they tried to use less *ghee* and butter, or substituted it with oil in order to reduce the risk of heart trouble. As will be shown later, it was the solid consistency of the fat that was seen to be the problem, and therefore solid vegetable products such as vegetable *ghee* (trade name Dalda) were identified as problematic in the same way as butter and butter-derived *ghee*.

The second hazard respondents identified with fat in the diet was that it led to weight gain which was a problem in and of itself and was connected to the increased risk of heart trouble. Fatty foods were said to be bad for health because they 'fill you up with grease and fat' and led to becoming overweight. Putting on weight was reported as leading to heart attacks, yet the precise nature of these links was not clear. Cholesterol, calories and fat were associated and, in fact, may almost be synonymous, since, for example, food that is 'bad' was described as 'probably very high calorie, lots of fat, lots of cholesterol, a really bad diet'. The synonymy of cholesterol and calories was such that a means of avoiding the problem of fattening food in the diet was to substitute Flora oil for butter in cooking. Changing from butter to a vegetable oil was thought to mean less cholesterol, fewer calories and therefore less of a fattening effect.

In order to avoid weight gain and heart trouble almost all respondents said that they were making an effort to eat less fatty food by avoiding fried items and using small amounts of oil in preparing other foods. The only exceptions were those women whose relationship with food was dominated by a medically diagnosed condition that they associated with thinness.

The foregoing discussion of the positive and negative health effects of food choice is clearly recognisable as a British, or more generally western, health promotion model: there are certain foods that are good, and should be featured in the diet; others contain bad constituents and lack good constituents, and should be avoided or eaten in moderation. In this reductionist model promotion and compromise of health were the key concepts in summing up the effect of different foods on the body. Women attributed the authority for this model to professional figures, such as teachers and doctors.

Notable by their absence were any expressions of disbelief in the dietary health beliefs of the reductionist type (cf. Frankel *et al.*

1991): possibly these may not have been expressed because the research project was affiliated to the general practice. It is not possible, therefore, to answer the question of whether young British Asian women treat reductionist-type dietary health beliefs with a scepticism similar to that to which their elders' systemic beliefs were subjected. Given their knowledge of British culture it seems likely that they would have similar criticisms to their non-Asian peers, but unlike their non-Asian peers they also have access to an alternative account of the relationship between food and health from which to construct criticism.

SYSTEMIC MODEL: MAINTAINING EQUILIBRIUM

Maintenance of equilibrium was the key concept in a different set of relations between health and food choice that featured in all respondents' accounts, and is referred to here as the systemic model. Rather than health being a quantum which could be added to or subtracted from by good or bad foods, health was viewed as an equilibrium that was dependent upon many different factors, only one of which was the food consumed, and the effect of each factor varied according to the other factors in operation. This synergistic model gives rise to a far more complex conception of the effect of food on health than the reductionist model.

In the systemic model the effect of food changed according to a number of factors: the way it was cooked and stored, the climate, the bodily state and stage of the life-cycle of the consumers, and sometimes their emotional state. A feature of these explanations was their reliance on some properties of food that are physical and can often be ascertained by lay people. For instance, accounts of the positive effects of *ghee* on constipation and stiff joints were understood to be due to its greasy quality which lubricates the body. Unlike the reductionist model, the authority of the systemic model derived from lay figures, mostly older relatives, especially mothers and mothers-in-law. Knowledge was acquired while growing up, 'from everyday use'. Unlike the authority of professionals, that of elders did not necessarily come from what they said so much as what they did.

The beliefs and practices that make up the systemic model were explained as common sense or as knowledge that has been passed on by relatives. Nevertheless, there are connections between the accounts in this study and the Ayurvedic and Unani healing systems, antecedents of which were being practised before the year 400 BC (or BCE, that is 'before the common era').[1] According to this tradition, disease causation is understood to be related to the imbalance of the biological humours or *dosas* of the body – air/wind, fire and phlegm/water – which determine the life processes of growth and decay (Frawley 1989: 4). An excess or deficiency of the humour can bring about various pathological changes in the body, the characteristics of which are related to the humour that is out of balance. Treatment for humoral imbalance is based on a system of tastes that apply to foods, minerals and herbs. This model is in contrast to the current orthodox western knowledge that views the onset of disease as the result of specific pathogens which invade an otherwise healthy body (Homans 1983: 174).

The humoral system as articulated in the traditions of Ayurveda and Unani is complex and highly developed, and only particular aspects of it appear in the accounts given by interviewees. The aspect most readily spoken of was heating and cooling, which has been identified as the element of a humoral system most likely to persist when others have been forgotten (Anderson 1984). The precise nature of the link between the science of Ayurveda and the understandings of health that are described is not covered in this chapter.

Heating and cooling were reported as having significant effects on the general health equilibrium and on particular symptoms. The heating and cooling effects of food were said to interact with the effects of the environment and the eater to influence health. In order to describe how this interactive system works some simplification is inevitable in what follows.

Cooling and heating foods

Although the effect of many foods was reported to vary according to the state of the person eating them and the climate, some were said to be particularly hot regardless of the context, including *karela* (Chinese prickly pear), meat, fish, eggs, chicken, nuts (particularly almonds) and garlic. There was said to be a connection between the way that foods were cooked and their heating effect; when cooked with dry heat and fat they become hotter in effect than if cooked with wet heat. Foods that were reported as having a particularly cooling effect included milk, okra, turnips, carrots, yoghurt, water, rice, *maash dahl* (unpolished orange lentils), oranges and ice cream. Consumption of these foods was said to affect the heat or coolness of the body, subject to other conditions, as described below.

The appearance, texture or taste of a food was said not to reveal its heating or cooling effect with any reliability. Some heating foods, such as ginger and garlic, could be identified by their distinctively strong or hot taste; they 'would taste bitter on your tongue, like nippy, like lemon juice, like vinegar'. But a strong taste was not viewed as a reliable guide to which foods were hot because there were also heating foods that did not have a burning or 'nippy' taste, and cooling foods that had a strong or bitter taste; for instance meat was reported to be heating, yet not to have a hot taste unless it is cooked with chillied spices. Meat was considered to have a strong heating effect independent of its taste. The heating effect of eating meat was compared to that of drinking a cup of tea, but to distinguish between hot temperature and hot effect on the body it was emphasised that although a cooked food could be hot in temperature, its effect on the body could still be cooling. The difficulty of distinguishing the heating effect of a food from thermal heat is shown in the following extract:

> they say it's just very warm for you. I'm not saying warm like sweating or whatever, not that sort of warm. I mean probably something inside that will affect you somewhere or other inside, but how I don't know.

Some heating foods were identified as such because they are rich in energy or protein, and this may be detected as a bodily sensation. For instance meat-eating was reported to impart a bodily sensation so that 'when you eat it, you feel inside you that you've got the goodness of it, like you've got the protein, the energy, from it' and a vegetable with a heating effect was 'very filling . . . it's rich'. It was claimed by some that the sensations when eating foods of different heating and cooling qualities were important because they offered the individual a guide to what should or should not be eaten in a particular season. Women who had grown up in the subcontinent were likely to claim that the interpretation of these sensations need not be learned, as the bodily sensations associated with being over-heated would automatically incline one towards cooling foods, whereas if one's body was over-cooled, heating foods would be desired. More serious disequilibrium was said to be signalled by distinct bodily and psychological symptoms. For instance, an excess of chilli was reported to lead to heartburn, too much fish can lead to a red swollen mouth, too much red meat can lead to a build up of anger and the general over-consumption of heating foods may result in pimples and itchy rashes. The question of whether changing bodily sensations in response to foods were thought to be inherent or culturally learned is discussed in more detail below when considering the plausibility that women attributed to this knowledge.

Foods with a cooling effect reportedly caused or exacerbated phlegmy, catarrhy conditions; they 'tend to put on a flu really quickly'. Cooling foods (together with other factors) were held responsible for exacerbating hacking coughs, flus and colds, and chest infections. Some of the foods that were said to exacerbate phlegmy conditions have themselves a mucus-like consistency, for instance yoghurt, or have the effect of creating mucus; for instance the phlegmy taste that is left in the mouth after drinking milk indicates a food that is particularly cooling. A food that has been warming can become cooling because of a change of consistency, for example *dahl* that has been left in the refrigerator for a few days takes on a glutinous, mucus-like feel and was said to have a more cooling effect than freshly-cooked *dahl*. Yet foods did not necessarily need to have a phlegmy consistency in order to encourage cold symptoms, since, for example, rice eaten during the winter was said to have similar effects to milk in promoting a chest infection.

In order to counter-act the cooling effects of these foods and prevent coldy, phlegmy symptoms, eating more warming foods was recommended. An informant whose family was strictly vegetarian (so not consumers of warming meat, eggs or fish), reported that she cooked a weekly dish of curry to which, in addition to the usual grated fresh ginger, she added *saunda*, a strong, dried ginger, whose potent heating effect offered extra protection from over-cooling during the winter months. Honey and tea made with raw grated ginger, both warming, were a preventive and a curative measure for colds, and honey could be rendered more warming, and therefore more effective at counter-acting a cold or other cooled condition, by adding 'quite a lot' of black pepper, before licking it from a spoon.

Climate and season

The weather was reported to make a difference to the heating or cooling effect of what was eaten, thus in Scotland's temperate, damp climate the maintenance of equilibrium requires a different strategy compared to what would be necessary in the hotter subcontinental climate. For the heating effect of some foods to be detrimental to health, the climate must be hot. During the subcontinental summer overheating was described as a serious risk and hence precautionary measures were a matter of urgency. In the summer in Pakistan, heating foods such as eggs and *karela* were forbidden, and the consumption of cooling foods such as boiled rice, *lassi* (yoghurt-based drink), yoghurt and milk were encouraged. In the winter in the subcontinent many of the cooling foods recommended in the summer, such as ice-cream, were not eaten, to avoid the possibility of over-cooling. Foods with a strong heating effect such as fish could be eaten to compensate for the cooling effect of the climate.

Precautions against over-heating were said not to apply in the summer in Scotland on the grounds that 'we don't usually get a summer', and consequently the possibility of climatic heat adding to the heating effect of a food was not considered a hazard. Although garlic, ginger and chillies were identified as very heating foods, it was stressed by respondents that in Britain they are eaten all the time according to taste and not season. Some people might moderate their intake of foods that are very heating in the summer in Scotland, but it was reported that the seasonal adjustments to their diets were minimal compared with Pakistan or India. The cool damp Scottish climate was said to be almost always over-cooling, especially in the winter. Precautions against this involved adding extra heat to the process of the consumption of a cooling foodstuff, either by heating the foodstuff or by heating the consumer through an external heat source or by giving them extra heating foods. These precautions were especially important for children and women of child-bearing age because of their particular vulnerability.

Life-cycle

Individuals' vulnerability to excesses of heating and cooling were said to vary during the life-cycle. Of concern to respondents was the increased vulnerability during childhood and, for women, at various stages in their reproductive careers, especially during menstruation and pregnancy. When young, children need protection from excesses of heating and cooling, so in Scotland many of the precautions described against over-cooling are applied with particular zeal to children. Some women said that their children were only ever given heated milk to drink in winter, and one mother insisted upon this in the summer too because of her daughter's tendency to catch colds. Children's intake of ice-cream and cold drinks was commonly reported to be strictly rationed, and one woman only allowed her children to consume such foods in front of a heater. Some children were given a spoon of honey (a heating food) every day after a meal during the winter months, and especially if they already had cold symptoms.

Although the temperate climate means that over-heating is not generally a concern in Scotland, children's greater vulnerability to extremes meant that precautions against over-heating were observed for them. A widespread belief, even amongst women who observed no other food avoidances, was that children should not be given too many eggs (a strongly heating food), otherwise nose bleeds and, for girls, the early onset of a heavy menstruation were likely to result. Chilli may have a similar effect on girls and should be given to children in modest amounts. The heating effect of nuts, equally, means that children's intake should be carefully rationed.

Pregnancy was regarded as a 'hot' state (see also Homans 1983), and therefore heating foods were proscribed during pregnancy to avoid 'too much heat for the body'. Menstruation was also identified as a 'warmed' state and so respondents recommended that heating foods, such as sultanas, should be avoided during 'monthlies', as should 'strongly cooked curries ... with lots of *masala* ... Indian pickles ... and sour foods like lemons'. Sour and pungent tastes are classified in Ayurveda as heating (Frawley 1989: 15). Eggs and fish are both heating foods and consumption of excess by menstruating women can lead to heavy periods, as illustrated by the following story, concerning an exchange between the speaker and her husband:

> the other day he had an egg in the morning and we were having fish and chips, fresh cod fillet in the evening and I says, 'Do you want a fried egg?' 'No', he says, 'Fish is hot and so is egg hot.

I don't want it.' I says, 'What you worried aboot? You're not gonnae get heavy periods!' . . . and he says, 'See you!'[2] and I says, 'Well, you asked for it, it was coming to you!'

If a woman wanted to precipitate a late period or bring on labour at the end of her pregnancy, intake of heating foods was recommended, for instance *saunda* (dried ginger powder) simmered with boiling water and drunk as a tea, or put into *dahl*. If taken during the early stages of pregnancy this type of hot food was said to lead to miscarriage. After childbirth, heating food is again prescribed to aid recuperation and strengthening of the mother's body. Traditionally the mother has a handful of *panjeeri* every day, which is a mixture of flour, *ghee*, sugar, nuts and sultanas which is said to be strongly heating, and helps her body to regain strength.

STATUS OF SYSTEMIC BELIEFS

By presenting the systemic understandings as an organised whole and in a written summary, it is easy to understate the dynamic, contingent way in which these beliefs are used in daily life in conjunction with other beliefs. Previous work on health beliefs of different ethnic groups has, at times, given the impression that to catalogue the reported effects of different foods on the body is to offer a complete understanding which permits prediction of consequent health behaviours (Thorogood 1990). Yet the current research shows that the context in which beliefs about heating and cooling are used is crucial to understanding their influence over health-relevant behaviours. Although the accounts of systemic beliefs were remarkably constant between all the respondents, there was variation as to the status that was accorded to the accounts.

Some women said that they avoided certain foods in certain seasons because they always had done so, without being able to report the reasoning behind the avoidances. Some claimed to have intuitive feelings about which foods were good for them on the basis of bodily sensations, others said they had no intuitive or bodily knowledge whatsoever, and what their mothers had told them was their only source of knowledge. The lack of bodily knowledge of the effects of food was often put down to having grown up in Scotland, with cold weather, so that eating too much heating food was almost impossible, and the feelings associated with over-heating were not experienced. Statements of disbelief in the heating and cooling effects of food were made by a minority of women, one of whom said 'That's a very Indiany thing to think about, you know', somewhat puzzled as to why it should be a topic in an interview about health. Women brought up in Britain and in the Indian subcontinent expressed disbelief, but they were nonetheless able to describe the systemic understandings of heating effects. They claimed that they often followed elders' recommendations on food consumption despite their stated disbelief.

Less harsh than disbelief was scepticism, which was expressed both by women who had been brought up in Britain and the Indian subcontinent alike; similarly, women whose elders were in Britain and the subcontinent reported that the latter also expressed disbelief in the ideas of heating and cooling. For instance, a woman cast mild doubt on her mother's advice: 'I think it's just what my mother tells me, yeah', and another suggested her elders' beliefs might be nothing more than superstition:

> I don't know what it's all about. Maybe it's just our superstition, I don't know, it seems to be true that everything is hot or cold.

A woman who followed her mother's habits and advice in avoiding certain foods at certain seasons said with assurance: 'I think we've all got it in our heads. . . . I think it's just what you believe in.' Sceptical women called their mothers' advice 'old ladies' tales from Pakistan', 'old days' tales', 'Granny Smith's tales' and 'myths' and could dismiss them as 'just more talk' from Pakistan. On specific issues such as eating *panjeeri* after childbirth, avoiding too many hot foods (e.g. almonds, boiled eggs, chicken and fish) or cold foods (e.g. ice-cream) under certain climatic conditions, women said that they knew their mothers had particular ideas, but they took no notice or 'didn't bother'. The *panjeeri* recommended for post-partum women, seemed to attract particular disdain from younger women as being 'old fashioned':

> *Answer*: Oh yes, *panjeeri*. Oh yes. . . . I never liked it. I can't stand the stuff. Oh right, yeah, that's really supposed to be good for you actually, 'cause it's got all the nuts and nutrients and everything in it.
> *Question*: But is that something that you eat at all?
> *Answer*: I hate that, that's so disgusting.

A cynical suggestion was that food prohibitions were 'probably an excuse or something' to stop children eating prized foods. This respondent then softened her attitude on the grounds, cited by many of the doubters, that she could not dismiss her parents' beliefs out of hand because they were so widespread: 'it's not only in my family; I've heard others saying it as well'.

There seems to be a contradiction between, on the one hand, widespread and often in-depth knowledge of Ayurvedic-type understandings of food and health, and, on the other hand, the expression of doubt over the veracity of these understandings. The first conclusion to be drawn from this contradiction is that a cautious approach should be taken towards the interpretation of the effects of reported systemic health beliefs on actual health behaviours. Second, in order for women to follow the advice of their mothers, they do not need to have a firm belief in the rationale behind the advice. If women's diets have been organised according to these principles since childhood, a strong reason would be necessary for them to reject familiar food habits. In the absence of strong evidence of ill effects, the safe course of action is to continue with familiar habits and the risky course is to reject them. Women preferred to trust their own mothers' experience and judgement, and to follow their advice, especially with children's diets, rather than place their children's health at risk. As one woman said, it is 'better to be safe than sorry'. Another commented that 'through experience the older generation know what's good and what's [not]', and so, she implied, why not benefit from their experience?

This conservatism in renouncing trusted elders' beliefs 'just in case' might account for the widespread nature of certain, specific health beliefs, such as the avoidance of eating fish and milk together. This combination was widely reported to give rise to a white skin rash, which one woman described as an eczema. Another woman explained that the rash had never been seen because no one would dream of mixing milk and fish:

> *Answer*: They say that you get some sort of white sting on your skin or whatever, I don't know what it is.
> *Question*: Have you ever seen that?
> *Answer*: No. Well, everybody avoids it.

Although some advice from elders was followed rigidly to be 'better safe than sorry', in cases where the risks involved are not too high, the advice could be put to the test. One respondent described how she tested the advice to avoid yoghurt with a cough and found that if she ate it she tended 'to cough even more that night, it does trigger it off' and 'makes it worse'. She concluded that the avoidance 'does help' and suggested that 'you don't *really* know until you try it'. Another woman found that she coughed or vomited up mucus if she ate cooling carrot, against her mother's advice to take warming meat or *dahl*, and therefore followed her mother's advice thenceforth. Yet, even if alternative authorities and experimentation showed elders' health advice to be apparently without foundation, it was still not necessarily always disregarded, especially for vulnerable groups such as children. One respondent reported having noted that fish and milk were cooked and eaten together in the hospital where she had her first child: 'I stayed in hospital and I used to get fish from there, they also used to give milk with it.' One of her English-speaking sisters-in-law had also discovered that their non-Asian general practitioner did not proscribe the consumption of fish and milk together. On the basis of this evidence of the acceptability to the medical profession of mixing milk and fish, she sometimes disregarded the injunction to avoid milk and fish together in her own diet, but for her children she was more cautious:

> Yes, for children I do take care, but if sometimes I have to drink [milk] then I drink. But for the children I take care in case something might happen.

On the occasions when young women reported disregarding their elders' advice, this could not necessarily be taken as evidence that they did not believe their elders. Advice and warnings might be believed, and while their veracity was not questioned, they were not heeded for different reasons. One woman reported that she chose not to follow her mother-in-law's warnings and was prepared to put up with the possibility of heavier periods as a result of eating 'too many hot things'. This woman acknowledged that her mother-in-law might be speaking the truth, and had her best interests at heart, but she valued her ability to eat preferred foods more highly than avoiding the risk of over-heating.

CONNECTIONS BETWEEN SYSTEMIC AND REDUCTIONIST ACCOUNTS

By presenting women's accounts of their health beliefs as belonging either to a systemic or a reductionist theory, which are contrasting in some respects, it might seem that these are mutually exclusive models of health. This was not the case, as women subscribed to both ways of thinking, and used one model to explain features of the other.

While accounts of challenges to reductionist recommendations based on systemic logic were not reported, there was some evidence that the former advice would only be followed insofar as it did not actually contradict traditional ways of understanding food and health. One instance was a woman who reported that: 'Nowadays mostly doctors say "Don't eat too much meat", or "Take white meat" or "Take more fish".' She confirmed that her family followed this advice and did eat fish instead of red meat, but not always. Fish is more strongly heating than meat, and this respondent's household liked to eat fish fried in a batter made with *besan* (flour made from ground yellow split peas) which renders it even more heating. Therefore they only followed the doctors' advice to eat more fish 'when it is more cold' because 'in summer we can't eat more of it because we don't have the taste for it'. Thus, while not challenging the logic of medical orthodoxy, this woman was explicit that she did not allow it to disrupt her alternative model.

One of the most powerful ways in which the two models of health could be tested was to explain the recommendations of one system in terms of the other. For example, butter and *ghee* were identified as 'bad' foods in the reductionist system and were connected with heart attacks. The necessity of moderating the intake of fatty foods was accepted by all respondents, but, as described earlier, the reductionist system did not explain why *ghee* and butter are implicated in increased risk of heart attacks. The systemic model could however compensate for this lack by focusing on the physical properties of fats. Fat, especially *ghee*, was reportedly 'good for your insides ... and your bones' because it provides lubrication, stopping them from getting dry which is particularly important if suffering from constipation or during childbirth.

This reasoning, in which reference was made to physical properties discernible by the respondent and affected by the climate, was extended to the explanation of the causes of heart attacks. It was explained that butter is solid at room temperature whereas oil is liquid. Foods cooked in butter solidify on cooling, particularly when put in the refrigerator, whereas those cooked with oil retain the liquid consistency that they have when hot. The health education and advertising that promotes using vegetable oils rather than animal-derived or dairy fats was understood to be because a similar process of solidification of the dairy fats happens inside the body, leading to blockages and therefore heart attacks, as explained below:

> I was told that it [Flora oil] is better than the *ghee*. The *ghee*, that's solid; it goes inside and sticks there. The liquids, that stays in a liquid. Even in winter the curry I make with Flora oil, it'll still be that I can spoon it out with something. If it's with *ghee* it'll go into a solid block and I can't separate it if I want a small portion out. So we've all changed to Flora oil. . . . The *ghee*, that's solid, it goes inside and sticks there.

Similarly:

> Those who are doing surveys say that butter is not good for your health because it is cold here so it gets jammed inside.

Butter 'jamming' or becoming stuck inside the body is a problem that was said to be more likely to occur in Scotland than in the subcontinent, because the weather is colder and therefore fats are more likely to solidify. This climatic element offered a means of explaining the fact that elders who grew up in the subcontinent 'were raised just eating butter', and attribute to it health-giving properties. The elders' beliefs in the positive effects of butter on health did not need to be denied by younger women, as they were seen to be pertinent to the subcontinental situation, but not Scotland. Thus a reductionist dietary recommendation was justified and explained by a systemic model, and in the process intra-generational differences in dietary health beliefs were accounted for.

A strengthening effect of foodstuffs was frequently cited as a reason for their inclusion in the diet and this effect was also expressed in the idiom of both the systemic and the reductionist systems. The reductionist advice suggested that egg, meat, vegetables, fruit, cheese and fish are full of protein and calcium and are therefore good for strong bones. The systemic strengthening effect was not attributed to a particular constituent such as protein, but was seen as part of the heating effect of foods that are highly calorific (Anderson 1984). Thus, evaporated milk on bread, *panjeeri* and a drink of milk with *ghee* and crushed almonds added were all recommended for building up strength, as was meat, which was widely regarded as very heating and also strengthening.

The heating and strengthening effect of meat is viewed as beneficial to health, but only within limits. Unlike vitamin-laden, fat-free fruit, meat does not have an absolute value in terms of health, and its benefits obey a law of diminishing returns. This is explicable in terms of both the systemic and the reductionist models. The reductionist warnings about over-consumption of meat concentrated on the fat that it might have on it, which could lead to overweight and cholesterol which 'your body doesn't need'. The systemic recommendation for moderation in meat consumption, in contrast, concerned the bodily problems of over-heating, such as rashes and pimples. Over-consumption of red meat was said sometimes to lead to emotional as well as physical imbalances, for instance a build up of *gussa* or anger.[3] The systemic and reductionist models thus agreed on the strategy for avoiding the ill effects of meat while still benefiting from its goodness, namely to eat plenty of vegetables with the meat and not eat it every day. One woman explained the biomedical dietary advice to increase the intake of vegetables without having to avoid meat altogether in terms of the sense of balance that is so crucial to the Unani/Ayurvedic understanding of health: 'Doctors say keep a balance; eat the right things. Eat vegetables too . . . go on eating meat but you should know about vegetables also.' Thus the case of meat, like that of butter and heart attacks, shows that it is possible for the two systems of thought to be brought to bear upon the same problem, and the consequent advice need not be viewed as conflicting.

CONCLUSION

Young Glaswegian women of Punjabi descent divide their daily foods into 'our foods' and 'their foods', both of which are featured in the daily diet. Health is a prime consideration in deciding upon the value of a food in the diet and there are two ways of judging its worth. The reductionist model rests on the authority of medical experts and explains the value of food in terms of its constituent parts and their effects on specific parts of the body, whereas the systemic or Ayurvedic model is derived from the advice of elders and takes a more contingent and interactive approach to assessing the merit of different foods in terms of an equilibrium. Great flexibility is demonstrated in the ways that the second model can be applied to explaining the health effects of different foods in different climates, at different points in the life-cycle and for different individuals. These two models are not viewed as being in competition with one another, but rather are used in a complementary fashion to compensate for one another's inadequacies. Used together the two models have considerable explanatory power to account for the connections between food and health that women encounter daily.

NOTES

1 Before the common era corresponds to the time prior to the birth of Jesus Christ. The common era or CE is equivalent to the years 'anno domini'. To refer to dates explicitly in terms of the birth of a Christian god seem particularly inappropriate in a study involving Sikhs, Muslims and Hindus.
2 'See you!' is a Glaswegian expression roughly equivalent to 'Hark at you!' or 'Look who's talking!'
3 The Ayurvedic system classifies emotions and consequent bodily states as hot (anger, ardour) or cold (calmness, impotence) and posits a link between these and the effect of food that is eaten (Jeffery et al. 1988: 24).

REFERENCES

Anderson, E.N. (1984) '"Heating and cooling" foods re-examined', Anthropology of Food 23, 415: 755–73.
Backett, K., Davison, C. and Mullen, K. (1994) 'Lay evaluation of health and healthy lifestyles: evidence from three studies', British Journal of General Practice 44: 277–80.
Bradby, H. (1996) 'Cultural strategies of young women of South Asian origin in Glasgow, with special reference to health', PhD Dissertation, Glasgow University, Glasgow.
Davison, C., Smith, G.D. and Frankel, S. (1991) 'Lay epidemiology and the prevention paradox: the implications of coronary candidacy for health education', Sociology of Health & Illness 13, 1: 1–19.
Frankel, S., Davison, C. and Smith, G.D. (1991) 'Lay epidemiology and the rationality of responses to health education', British Journal of General Practice 41: 428–30.
Frawley, D.D. (1989) Ayurvedic Healing, Delhi: Motlilal Banarsidass.
Helman, C.G. (1990) Culture, Health and Illness, London: Wright.

Homans, H. (1983) 'A question of balance: Asian and British women's perceptions of food during pregnancy', in A. Murcott (ed.) *The Sociology of Food and Eating: Essays on the Sociological Significance of Food*, Aldershot: Gower.

Jeffery, P., Jeffery, R. and Lyon, A. (1988) *Labour Pains and Labour Power*, London: Zed Books.

Thorogood, N. (1990) 'Caribbean home remedies and their importance for black women's health care in Britain', in P. Abbott and G. Payne (eds) *New Directions in the Sociology of Health*, Basingstoke: Falmer Press.

Chapter 12

Scaremonger or scapegoat?

The role of the media in the emergence of food as a social issue

Jacquie Reilly and David Miller

Discussion about the reporting of food risks is peppered with criticisms of the media, which are variously blamed for purveying the 'propaganda' of the food industry or the government, or promoting unhealthy foods. Alternatively, the media are alleged to damage sales, to be anti-business, a source of unwarranted scares and in the grip of the food 'fascists',[1] 'terrorists'[2] or 'Leninists'.[3] In all cases the media are seen as irresponsible and sensationalist, either by uncritically allowing the nation's health to be damaged by the food industry or causing undue alarm by publicising the views of non-experts, pseudo-scientists and politically motivated pressure groups.

This chapter[4] will draw attention to three main problems with these explanations:

1 Media organisations are not independent. Instead they are heavily dependent on their sources for information and context.
2 Media institutions are treated as though they are homogeneous, whereas in fact different media (and different parts of a single medium) have distinct and sometimes contradictory interests.
3 The impact of the media is not always predictable from an examination of media content alone.

These points will be illustrated by referring to some of the food risk stories which have arisen over the last few years, and by looking more specifically at BSE (bovine spongiform encephalopathy) or 'Mad Cow Disease'.

MEDIA SOURCES AND THEIR STRATEGIES

Media institutions depend for their existence on their sources. Without informants there would be very little of what we currently understand as news. One consequence of focusing attention on the media as the cause of many and diverse social ills is that critics often lose sight of the relationship between the media and other social institutions in the production of news accounts. News sources increasingly recognise the value of planning media strategies to deal with their image in the media and with the public. For example, the Department of Health (DoH) and the Ministry of Agriculture (MAFF) employ large numbers of information officers whose function is to liaise between the media and the department. These government departments are the continuous site of bureaucratic activity which produce large amounts of information for journalists every day. Such institutions have a considerable potential for managing news coverage in ways favourable to themselves.

However, if media strategies contain diverse elements which pull against each other then contradictions within strategies, should they emerge, will obviously be news. It is in this sense that we can speak of media strategies being well or poorly handled. The concern about Patulin in apple juice in 1993 is a case in point. There seems to have been a feeling in some parts of MAFF that the handling of that incident was a case of the Ministry shooting itself in the foot. The story reached the media in February 1993, but the contamination had been known about for seven months and had deliberately been kept from the public. Much of the press concern at the time was about what was seen as unacceptable secrecy in MAFF which had been promoting itself, quite successfully, as the most open department in Whitehall. Indeed in an interview with the *Guardian* in January 1993, the Food Minister Nicholas Soames had gone so far as to claim that 'It's impossible to give the brutes more. If the Chief Vet does have a secret file stuck up his jumper, I don't know about it' (2.1.1993), while at the same time, his department was sitting on information about poisoned apple juice.

Government, industry and pressure groups all recognise the value of formulating strategies to gain influence, and many such strategies will include a media dimension. Indeed, any organisation which attempts to manage the media will find itself in competition with a whole range of others in its own field and beyond for space and favourable comment. Sometimes media strategies will involve explicit aims in relation to competition or co-operation with other organisations. The National Farmers Union, for example, has, since 1990, instituted a three-phase Public Affairs strategy which located some of the problems of the farming industry in the 'siege mentality' of farmers themselves (Dillon 1990). Two years later, the NFU themselves regarded the strategy as a great success, described in an internal report in the following terms: 'The *Today* programme, one of the most influential among decision-makers, has now made it official: "Farmers are no longer whingeing"' (Dillon Roberts 1992). Thus the planning of such strategies recognises that it is necessary and potentially possible to improve relations with the media and hence that problems of image or power are not only due to the media themselves.

Bureaucratic organisations do, of course, house large numbers of competing interests and agendas, and it is precisely the function of the press office to manage such differences and potential divisions and present a unified face to the outside world (Miller 1993, Miller and Williams 1993), since a divided organisation can be a weak one. Similarly a divided government can mean either the failure of government agenda-building or conversely the success of one part of government in promoting its own interests at the expense of others. It is too simplistic to say that such divisions are then reported or exaggerated by the media. In fact media interest in such divisions is an intimate part of the failure.

For instance, one of the key factors which prompted the explosion of interest in salmonella in eggs in early December 1988 was an obvious division within government between the DoH and MAFF. The rise in salmonella poisoning and the attempts by MAFF and the industry to keep it out of the news was well documented by the Commons Agriculture Committee in their report *Salmonella in Eggs* (1989a, 1989b). After Edwina Currie had made her famous statement that 'Most of the egg production in this country, sadly, is now infected with Salmonella', the media interest could not be sustained under its own momentum and the 'story' would in fact have died a lot sooner than it did, had it not been for an abrupt tactical about-turn by the industry, including the National Farmers Union. Instead of playing the issue down, the strategy at the NFU was to keep it in the news in order to push for compensation and to secure Edwina Currie's departure.

The story was eventually limited not only by Edwina Currie's resignation but also by a shift in media coverage of perceptions of the cause of the problem from egg production to kitchen hygiene. Speaking very generally, this is one reason why salmonella is different to the issue of BSE (bovine spongiform encephalopathy) which has not been dampened so quickly. Indeed, the very uncertainty of scientific knowledge on BSE has meant that the topic can continue to re-emerge regularly on the front pages of the newspapers.[5]

Divisions in scientific knowledge can also lead to controversies in the media especially if new research appears to overturn scientific orthodoxy. Journalism relies on credible, authoritative and expert sources since journalists have no independent set of criteria by which to evaluate the truth of news stories. Natural science, by contrast, does claim to have an independent way of knowing the truth about the world. In fact, as Anne Karpf has pointed out 'science and medicine still have a unique social authority, as if they somehow by-pass social, political, economic and emotional factors: we seem to believe that science is thought with the thinkers removed – as if that were possible' (Karpf 1993). So, when apparently reputable and high-status research gives new and controversial findings, it is difficult for journalists to ignore. Nonetheless, some journalists do have quite explicit positions on debates and hence new research is more or less welcome in accordance with such positions.

MEDIA AGENDAS AND THEIR IMPACT

Media institutions are not simply the instruments of either government, the food industry or of pressure groups: they too have their own interests and agendas. Newspapers are run as a business, but this does not mean that they simply go for the story which will bring in the most readers: they are carefully targeted at particular social groupings, and stories will thus, to some extent, reflect the 'personality' of the paper. Furthermore, despite recent changes in broadcasting regulation, television and radio do still retain a significant public service ethos, albeit in retreat, which can mean that some sections of the broadcast media consider their role as an educative one.

Media organisations can themselves be highly internally differentiated. The work of one journalist or producer can result in reports or programmes which are completely contradictory in factual details or in perspective to that of another. In the broadsheet press there are a large number of specialist correspondents who each have their own 'beats' and their own range of contacts. Health and medical correspondents have quite different contacts from those covering agriculture and these in turn are different from consumer correspondents. Specialist journalists can often become very close to their sources and dependent on a limited range of contacts, for example, in the post-war period *The Times* agriculture correspondent was, according to Martin Smith, 'almost a member of the policy community'.[6]

The increase in the coverage of food issues in the last ten years is also partly attributable to the marketing strategies of newspapers. In the 1970s food writing in the broadsheets was largely confined to what has been called the 'ghetto' of the women's pages: 'The usual dose then was a weekly cookery column from a single regular, outside contributor' (Crawford-Poole 1993: 19). In contrast, from being a domestic topic appearing weekly on the women's page, food and drink writing now has its own two- or three-page spread in the style and leisure parts of the weekend paper. Such an increase in food writing opportunities resulted in the formation in April 1984 of the Guild of Food Writers (Cooper 1985) which sees itself as having a campaigning agenda; since 1989 it has produced its own newsletter. One consequence of this process has been the opening up of space in the food pages for critical and political views on food as well as just recipes and gourmet writing.

The existence of advertising is an additional factor in newspapers and on commercial television, since its content is determined (within certain limits) by the motive of selling products. This is quite different from a public service motivation and means that there can often be a contradiction between the messages given about food in advertising and those in editorial coverage. However, given that advertising revenue is what funds commercial television, there is a sense in which, as Golding and Murdock have argued, it is audiences themselves rather than television programmes which are the primary commodity. They note that: 'The economics of commercial broadcasting revolves around the exchange of audiences for advertising revenue' (1991: 20). So the need to secure large audiences promotes the production of familiar programming and limits the production of innovative or risky programmes.

'Hence the audience's position as a commodity serves to reduce the overall diversity of programming and ensure that it confirms established mores and assumptions far more often than it challenges them' (Golding and Murdock 1991: 20). The contest between food and health pressure groups and advertisers over acceptable advertising is thus adjudicated on by a body (the Independent Television Commission) which, although required by law to be 'independent', depends for its existence on advertising revenue (see Dibb 1993 for some decisions on particular cases).

The main debates about the problems of the media revolve around their damaging impact on the 'gullible' public. What we should also realise is that the media can have effects on industry, government, pressure groups and a host of other categories of organisation. It seems likely, for instance, that the Food Safety Act was born partially out of media coverage of salmonella and listeria. Similarly a high media profile can bring in new resources or membership for poorly resourced pressure groups. Often the results of media coverage on policy or politics will not be visible to the general public but will make important differences to the organisations involved.

A major problem for critics of the malign influence of the media is their assumption that the impact of the media is straightforward and direct. Consumers, especially children and other groups perceived as vulnerable, are thought to be particularly at risk from media messages, whether emanating from health education literature or advertising (Dibb 1993, Karpf 1990). The problem is that people do not passively absorb everything that is beamed from their television set. Instead they interpret and contextualise. They might end up believing the information they get from television or the press or advertising, or they might not.

In the next section, we discuss in some detail the media coverage of BSE, the reasons why it developed as it did, and some of the relationships between promotional strategies, media coverage and policy outcomes.

SCAREMONGER OR SCAPEGOAT: THE CASE OF BSE

The story of BSE is an extremely complex one, much of which has become the subject of extensive media coverage itself (see Miller and Reilly 1994, 1995), stretching back to 1985 when the first cases were diagnosed. The main debate has centred on the science of BSE and whether, through contamination via infected bovine products, it can be passed to humans. There has always been a theoretical risk that BSE could be transmitted in this way, but while many 'experts' on the subject have admitted to this possibility (however unlikely or remote they believed it to be), the government has tended to maintain the message: 'There is no risk to humans.' The Southwood Committee set up by the government in April 1988 to assess the significance of the new disease reported that 'the risk of transmission of BSE to humans appears remote and it is unlikely that BSE will have any implications for human health'. But it also added: 'If our assessments of these likelihoods are incorrect, the implications would be extremely serious . . . with the long incubation period of spongiform encephalopathies in humans, it may be a decade or more before complete reassurances can be given' (Southwood 1989). However, in the subsequent joint MAFF/DoH press release the qualifying clauses were left out: 'the report concludes that the risk of transmission of BSE to humans appears remote and it is therefore most unlikely that BSE will have any implications for human health' (*BBC News* 21.00, 27.2.89).

From the beginning of the affair in 1985, MAFF tried to control all aspects of communication on BSE. It was not until June 1986 (seven months after the first diagnosis) that it informed ministers of the new outbreak and a further ten months elapsed before the government moved to have the threat assessed.

When MAFF finally announced the existence of the new disease it did so in the 'Short Communications' section of the *Veterinary Record* (journal of the British Veterinary Asssociation). This was picked up by the *Daily Telegraph* (25.10.87), *The Times* (29.12.87) and on *BBC News* (30.10.87), with the reporting centred on a potentially threatening cattle disease. No mention was made of the possibility of an extended host range which could include humans.

In July 1988, John McGregor (then Minister of Agriculture) stopped the feeding of cattle and sheep brains and offal to cattle and sheep. Inevitably, the next question to be asked was about human food. While animals were no longer eating the specified offals, there was no such legislation for humans. Pre-clinical BSE cattle were still going into the national food chain as if they were healthy animals, with brains, spinal cord, spleen, thymus, tonsils, intestines and bits of spinal tissue being used in 'mechanically recovered meat' in a variety of products such as burgers, meat pies, pâtés, lasagne, soups, stock cubes and baby foods. By March 1989 McGregor was asked to ban human consumption of any organs known to harbour infectious agents. He at first refused on the grounds that it was 'not appropriate' but this was finally done in November 1989. — B.V.O BAN .

Pressure mounted for more to be done and the farming community demanded 100 per cent compensation for the destruction of its animals. By 1989, other countries began to be interested in the disease: Australia had already banned British beef cattle exports in July 1988. It was not, however, until Germany announced its intention to ban UK beef, unless it was accompanied by a certificate proving that the meat had originated from BSE-free herds, that BSE was catapulted from a worrying cattle problem into an international crisis.

In fact, media coverage of BSE developed slowly, and did not enter mainstream public debate until 1990. There was already a well-developed interest in food safety because of salmonella and listeria, and the government was in the process of introducing a new Food Safety Act. Food had been in the media throughout 1988 and 1989, but BSE had been hidden behind the other so-called 'food scares', coming to prominence only when political actors engaged with the issue. In that year the number of cases of BSE began rising rapidly, reaching 14,000 officially confirmed cases by the end of the year. Germany, Italy and France all banned British beef imports. In Britain the death of a domestic cat from a spongiform encephalopathy caused further alarm, opening the debate on transmission and bringing the potential threat to humans a little closer. Local councils banned beef from the menus of 2,000 schools. The farming community and the meat industry again applied pressure on the government to do something, but the government only issued guidelines on BSE to farmers in May 1990, five years after the initial diagnosis of the disease, and it was not until February 1991 that the farmers started to receive 100 per cent compensation.

The tight control over information ultimately allowed the story of BSE to develop in a particular direction by opening the way for different players actively to engage with the media, to establish positions of credibility, to debate and ask questions. It also meant that the account of the nature and extent of the risks of BSE offered by the government was contested and subject to redefinition.

Yet processes at work both at the level of the production of scientific assessments and within the media meant that voices arguing that beef was unsafe were to some extent muted. One such factor involved MAFF's influence over the scientific debate itself: keeping public health out of the debate, attempting to control the research, to define who were seen as 'experts' and to limit what people were allowed to say in public (see Miller and Reilly 1996).

HOW THE STORY WAS MANAGED

Until recently MAFF has kept public health interests out of the decision-making process by stressing that BSE was essentially a veterinary problem with no risks to human health. Those involved in public health have concurred in this. The press release of February 1989 which stated that BSE held only a 'remote risk' to human beings was jointly produced by MAFF and the DoH. MAFF apparently used its influence to reduce research in the Public Health Laboratory, the body responsible for monitoring communicable diseases. As a source within the Public Health Laboratory Service said during interview:

> We were told that we had to send everything to MAFF. Everybody wanted to know why, I mean it was obvious to us that this was a public health issue. But no, apparently it wasn't, we couldn't believe it. We were all ready to move on this thing and then we had to stop. The word from above was that it was MAFF's thing . . . and we had to hand over everything to them. There was absolutely nothing we could do about it.[7]

MAFF also influenced who were seen as the main experts in the field through, for example, appointments to the various committees which were established. These were the people likely to be called on for comment, and trusted, by specialist journalists. However, their expertise was challenged from outside government circles:

> Those of us in the field realised that the small group of people in SEAC (the Spongiform Encephalopathy Advisory Committee) included only a few who understood the subject fully (and even they were known to believe that BSE was a minor risk). For example, one of the members was a vet, another an expert in foot and mouth disease, another a histologist, another

a retired manager of a veterinary research laboratory. Even the chairman had been an expert on the common cold. Yet the government was making it clear to the press that these were the national experts on the subject of BSE and that they were taking their advice from them.

(Dealler 1996)

MAFF also tried to control what was said in public in order to minimise the possibilities of public alarm (and the repercussions this might bring). What has become clear is that while the public was being told that BSE couldn't get into food, and even if it could it wouldn't do any harm, there was real concern being expressed by scientists. Worry intensified as animals other than cattle – first antelopes, then cats, then pigs – succumbed. As Professor Jeff Almond, a member of the government advisory committee (SEAC) said on a TV documentary:

The more animal species that became affected, the more one worried about the transmissibility potential of BSE and the possibility that it would include humans. There's no getting away from that.

(*Panorama* 17.6.96)

In early 1989, the official government view was that the removal of offals from human food was completely unnecessary but in May of that year Hugh Fraser, one of the most senior researchers at the Institute of Animal Health, said on Radio 4's *Face the Facts* that he no longer ate bovine offals, and that it would be prudent if suspect tissues were removed from human consumption. As a result:

I and senior colleagues were told not to discuss these matters with the media, and that if media questions arose they should be diverted elsewhere. And although the Ministry of Agriculture were probably aware of the things that I was talking about, they preferred to manage the way in which this was presented and dealt with.

(*Panorama* 17.6.96)

More recently, in 1995, neuropathologist Sir Bernard Tomlinson attracted a great deal of media attention when he said, again on a Radio 4 programme, that all beef offal should be banned for human consumption. Tomlinson's statements might have gone unnoticed had press releases not been organised and mainstream TV and print media made aware of what he had said – that there was a risk from offals which were still being used in human food.[8]

MEDIA FACTORS WHICH MUTED THE STORY

There have been long periods of time when BSE has not been deemed 'newsworthy'[9] and therefore could not be sustained on a day-to-day level in news terms. Coverage has peaked, not randomly, but in relation to a complex interaction between science, government policy decisions (both British and international), secrecy and public responses to reporting.

One factor is that while government inaction can cause uproar, this will tend to die down when officials are seen to be doing something about the issue in question. This is perfectly clear when we see how BSE began to disappear from the media agenda once Britain had some success in stopping the European bans on beef in 1990. The same thing occurred following the reporting of CJD (Creutzfeld-Jakob disease) cases in 1992.

A second factor is the way the media themselves operate. Unless a feature or column is being prepared the majority of reporting will come from press releases or articles in scientific journals, sources which the media use heavily, and thus the actual reporting of BSE does not necessarily mirror the incidence or severity of the disease. While media coverage of BSE all but disappeared for some time after 1990/1, the disease did not go away and the threat of human transmission remained the big unanswered question.

Although a number of journalists have always remained intensely interested in the subject, they have often fallen foul of editorial decision-making and the demands of hard news. As one broadsheet correspondent commented:

> It's logical really. Newspapers demand new information, new angles, controversy what have you. I couldn't get BSE in all the time. They lost interest in the subject because nothing was happening. Of course that was the whole point, nothing was happening to destroy this thing, but in newspaper terms I wouldn't be given the space to say that every day or every week. At the same time a few of us were seen as being slightly OTT on the subject, a bit nutty. I don't think people really believed that there was a real danger from beef – there were no

dead people (at that time) so, in a sense, although I was given a lot of scope, what had to happen for the full-scale go-ahead of a major story was dead people. Well, we've got them now.[10]

The 'experts' had never encountered this disease in cattle before, and therefore did not know how it would develop. Scientists could make predictions, and were encouraged to do so because of a lack of official information. As one broadsheet journalist said:

> Basically, because scrapie had been a disease that nobody cared about, the scientists in the subjects were the oddballs of the world. All very nice, but there was only going to be one Nobel Prize from this and they were determined to disagree with each other. This meant that if you wanted to find someone to say that BSE was not a risk, well that was fairly easy, but if you wanted people to say that BSE should be avoided like the plague then that was easy too.[11]

Government officials and scientists given leave to speak to the media have been very careful about what they say, but dissenting voices have always been in existence and, on occasion, entered the public debate. The most audible has been that of Richard Lacey. Variously dubbed a 'prophet of doom', a 'charlatan' and a 'sensationalist', Lacey has been a thorn in the side of official pronouncements of risk since the beginning of the BSE crisis. From 1989 he has said that it could infect humans, could pass from cow to calf, and that because the disease was not adequately understood, the potential risks demanded that the slaughter of cattle herds should take place to destroy it once and for all.

> I can see no alternative but to eliminate all the infected herds, because it is not possible to identify which animal is infected before it gets a terminal illness. An infectious agent could be brewing up months or years before the animal becomes ill. So, I see no way of detecting this. . . . I can't see any other way but the most unpleasant prospect of elimination of a large number of cattle in this country.
>
> (*BBC1 News* 21.00, 14.5.90)

His style was attractive in terms of controversy, so, for example, the above statement was translated on to the front page of *The Sunday Times* as 'a report stating that the risks of humans catching "mad cow" disease were so great that six million cattle had to be slaughtered' (*The Sunday Times* 13.5.90).

MAFF firmly rejected Lacey's views on risk, and, while certain parts of the media were attracted by his statements, what he said was (in political terms) easily discredited. A broadsheet journalist commented that they couldn't report what he said beyond a certain point because:

> Lacey was right all along. But he couldn't prove it so MAFF always won the argument. 'Bring us your evidence' they'd say. Of course, it was pretty hard to get any when they controlled everything. But he was a scientist saying the opposite to what the government experts – scientists as well – were saying so he could be written off as the sort of lone prophet of the apocalypse. It was easy for them really, everything he said was so extreme in relation to the calm, consistent way that the government had developed their statements about safety, using expert science and the best independent advice line. And he looked a bit mad too.[12]

However, Lacey and others were not totally discredited in the media and the issue did rumble on at a certain level. In some ways it was precisely the official silence on the topic and attempts to control information which facilitated this, which brings us to the fourth factor in the development of the story. This is that official silence led to a news vacuum, and different interest groups actively engaged with the media in an attempt to influence the debate and policy.

Because MAFF attempted to keep such tight control over information on BSE and CJD, alternative media sources were found and 'experts' created. Behind the scenes, sources used by the media would be scientists, researchers and organisations such as the British Veterinary Association (Miller and Reilly 1995). In this way those journalists who consistently covered the story were writing from a well-researched point of view, and could ask questions which were not being asked at other levels. Their highlighting of conditions and practices within slaughterhouses, for example, changed the issue from one of whether bovine offals were being removed to one of how effectively or safely this was being done. An Environmental Health Office (EHO) document sent to MAFF in February 1990 had pointed out that poor practices were evident. They received no reply from the Ministry. It

has only been since 1995 (six years after the directive) that MAFF
has taken steps to tighten controls on slaughterhouse practices.
Had the media not brought research into poor hygiene and clear
breaches of regulations into the open then work by, for example,
the EHO, might have gone unnoticed. A member of the Institute
of Environmental Health Officers said:

> It did help. We approached certain journalists and said, 'Look
> we've found out that there are some disgracefully risky things
> going on in abattoirs, and something has to be done about it.
> Will you print it?' The good ones . . . agreed. Now while that
> would have happened eventually, with government it is neces-
> sary to get the ball rolling, everything takes such a long time. But
> if there is public concern that can move things along . . . and with
> BSE the government were so paranoid about not being seen to
> be doing something that they reacted pretty damn quickly. It's
> not the ideal way of doing things, but when needs must . . . [13]

Undoubtedly media attention has in this way influenced policy
on BSE: the media have been used to force the government to 'go
public'. For example, Lacey and colleagues decided early on that
the only way to get BSE onto the agenda in 1989 was to go to the
media, particularly the foreign press. To put BSE firmly on the
British political agenda, concern had to come from outside.
According to one researcher:

> What came from all this was the fact that the media were the
> most efficient and effective way of getting anything done. . . .
> MPs could not understand, government organisations had
> been told to do nothing . . . there was a consensus of ignorance
> among the medical profession and large numbers of experts
> who did not say anything, even though they knew the risk was
> bad. So, the media were the only route by which information
> could reach the public . . . [14]

Following the major crisis of 1990, official statements on BSE
continued to insist that there was no risk to humans. Then came a
Department of Health statement on 20 March 1996, when Stephen
Dorrell announced the existence of a new strain of the human
disease CJD and the possibility of a link with BSE, which was seen
to be the most likely explanation for the new strain of CJD. This
re-ignited the long-running controversy over the safety of British
beef for a number of reasons.

First of all, while clear pronouncements about safety were being made to the public, new CJD cases had started to appear in 1994, when there were six, and continued in 1995, by which time ten cases had appeared in younger people. According to the chair of SEAC, John Pattison, projected cases of BSE in humans, calculated on current information, were seen as potentially representing a major public health problem, and so the committee decided that the news had to be made public.

Going public with information on a new strain of CJD has changed the nature of the BSE debate, so that human health interests have finally been brought into play. Even so, while SEAC made recommendations that the risk to humans from food would probably be small if there were better controls on offals and more rigorous enforcement of those controls, John Major was seen on TV saying that beef was 'entirely safe' and that this had been confirmed by British scientists (*PM* 23.4.96)

Second, the media has reported on people who have died or are dying at an early age, with pictures of those suffering from CJD, and interviews with their families. A pressure group member described what it was like to see the effects of the disease:

> You look at the pictures of Vicky Rimmer or Peter Hall, both just kids for God's sake, and you think 'How could this happen to people like that?' I was totally distressed, and I know a lot of other people who were too. Then there are the mothers, who are so confused and guilty, blaming themselves because it was them who fed their children this risky food. They believe it was meat which caused it, for the simple reason that scientists and doctors who have been testing their kids cannot come up with any other explanation. I met the CJD support group and it was one of the most profound experiences I've ever had. To be staring death in the face so blatantly without being able to do a damn thing about it . . . then to be told by those on high that you are wrong. Well, it makes people angry, and [they] want action. They will use any means, including what must be painful interviews in the media, to get their point across. And I think to some extent it has worked, an impact has been made. We now have so many calls from people, who, having seen *Panorama* or whatever, are shocked, and want to know what to do.[15]

The third factor which brought the disease to the forefront in 1990, 1992 and again in 1996 was European intervention.

European countries claimed they were protecting the public health but in 1990 John Gummer treated this view as one of powerful vested interests playing at protectionism, aided by 'media hype and sensationalism'. He issued what could only be described as a call to arms, asking that we all, 'including the BBC, ITN and others', refuse to let the European Community control Britain. In spite of this, the opinion which was currently most clearly articulated in media coverage in 1996 was that the development of BSE was largely the fault of the British government.

CONCLUSION

BSE is likely to remain a media story as long as scientific uncertainties remain about the cause of new CJD cases and, as a consequence, as long as European intervention ensures that there are controls on beef exports. Our argument has been that the media have been shown in this paper to provide an arena in which contests for definition take place. Although undoubtedly that arena is uneven and there is structured inequality of access to it, nevertheless contest does take place, as the media provide information to the public and are the focus of strategies by many groups. It is therefore important to go beyond media-centric explanations and understand that the way in which the media operates is a product of complex interactions between media, the social institutions on which they report and the public.

NOTES

1 As then Agriculture Minister John Gummer has dubbed those who are 'spreading unwarranted alarm about the safety of British food'. (See Michael Hornsby, 'Gummer attack on food alarmists', *The Times* and 'Gummer blasts food "fascists"', *Daily Star* 1.2.90.)
2 See e.g. 'The food terrorists are on the attack once again', in Egon Ronay, 'Eat up your greens – the food fascists are on the march again', *The Sunday Times* (8.3.92).
3 See e.g. 'Don't panic, it's only a paranoia of food Leninists', *Glasgow Herald* (28.1.92).
4 This chapter arises from two research projects, 'The Role of the Media in the Emergence of Food Panics' as part of the ESRC-funded Nation's Diet programme (grant L209252011)and 'Media and Expert Constructions of Risk', funded under ESRC's Risk and Human Behaviour programme (grant L211252010).
5 By comparison salmonella is a dead issue. Our database of press

coverage of food issues contains 104 news stories on BSE for the year 1992. By comparison there are a mere 13 on salmonella in the same period. Unless it can be shifted back to a problem of production salmonella is unlikely to become a major issue again.

6 Conversation with Martin Smith, Department of Politics, Sheffield University, 29.4.88. (See also Smith 1989, 1991.)

7 Interview with one of the authors, November 1995.

8 One example of how media treatment of BSE attracted attention came with the drama programme 'Natural Lies' in 1992. MAFF intervened in the programme because they were worried it would generate public fears and harm beef sales. In 1992 media coverage of BSE had declined to such an extent that there were only 94 national press items (15 of which were TV reviews of the drama itself), as opposed to 1,092 items in 1990. But the level of concern from MAFF about its re-emergence is clear when they attempt to influence TV drama. John Gummer contacted the BBC because the expert advisers being used on the programme were Helen Grant and Richard Lacey (*Observer* 24.5.92). While the programme did go on the air, the BBC did make changes. For example, one statement in the series, 'I believe one man has died from the virus' was re-recorded as 'A man may have contracted BSE even faster through an open wound'.

9 For example, in 1990 there were 1,092 national newspaper articles on BSE as compared with 93 in 1991.

10 Interview with one of the authors, April 1996.

11 Interview with one of the authors, January 1996.

12 Interview with one of the authors, July 1995.

13 Interview with one of the authors, April 1994.

14 Interview with one of the authors, May 1995.

15 Interview with one of the authors, July 1996.

REFERENCES

Commons Agriculture Committee (1989a) *Salmonella in Eggs*, First Report, Report and Proceedings of the Committee, Vol. 1, 28 February.

—— (1989b) *Salmonella in Eggs*, First Report, Minutes of Evidence and Appendices, Vol. 2, 28 February.

Cooper, Derek (1985) 'A new voice', *The Listener* 7 November: 17.

Crawford-Poole, Shona (1993) 'Consuming fashions', *The Guild of Food Writers News* 9, Spring: 19.

Dealler, Stephen (1996) *Fatal Legacy: BSE, the Search for the Truth*, London: Corgi.

Dibb, S. (1993) *Children: Advertisers' Dream, Nutrition Nightmare?* London: National Food Alliance.

Dillon, Anne (1990) *Public Affairs Strategy*, June, London: National Farmers Union.

Dillon Roberts, Anne (1992) *Public Affairs Strategy 3*, October, London: National Farmers Union.

Golding, Peter and Murdock, Graham (1991) 'Culture, communications and political economy', in James Curran and Michael Gurevitch (eds) *Mass Media and Society*, London: Edward Arnold.

Karpf, Anne (1990) *Doctoring the Media: The Reporting of Health and Medicine*, London: Routledge.

—— (1993) 'On medical journalism', *Observer Magazine*, 15 August: 45.

Miller, David (1993) 'Official sources and primary definition: the case of Northern Ireland', *Media, Culture & Society* 15 (3): 385–406.

Miller, David and Reilly, Jacquie (1994) *Food 'Scares' in the Media*, Glasgow: Glasgow University Media Group.

—— (1995) 'Making an issue of food safety: the media, pressure groups and the public sphere', in Donna Maurer and Jeffrey Sobal (eds) *Food, Eating and Nutrition as Social Problems: Constructivist Perspectives*, New York: Aldine De Gruyter.

—— (1996) 'Mad cows and Englishmen', Planet: The Welsh Internationalist 117 (June/July): 118–19.

Miller, David and Williams, Kevin (1993) 'Negotiating HIV/AIDS information: agendas, media strategies and the news', in Glasgow University Media Group, *Getting the Message*, London: Routledge.

Smith, Martin J. (1989) 'Changing agendas and policy communities: agricultural issues in the 1930s and the 1980s', *Public Administration* 67: 149–65.

—— (1991) 'From policy community to issue network: salmonella in eggs and the new politics of food', *Public Administration* 69: 235–55.

Southwood, R. (1989) *Report of the Working Party on Bovine Spongiform Encephalopathy*, London: HMSO.

Chapter 13

Declining meat

Past, present . . . and future imperfect?

Nick Fiddes

INTRODUCTION: THE WIDENING OF THE ETHICAL NET

Moral values habitually cast as absolute and eternal are demonstrably anything but: *what* is seen as morally acceptable can and does vary enormously between individuals, places and periods. Perhaps as crucially, the definition of those regarded as 'like ourselves' and so deserving of consideration, is seldom a simple matter. When, amid an epidemic of BSE publicity, stories spread of Indian Hindus offering sanctuary to British cattle threatened with culling, the British media responded mainly with facetious amusement at such sentimentality towards beasts.

Meditating on moral systems' transience might seem a convenient departure point for some postmodernist treatise on meat's contemporary crisis of identity, as evidenced by its turbulent reputation in terms of both health and compassion, and manifested in dramatically fluctuating sales amid significant long-term decline. But, perhaps paradoxically, there are also good reasons to suppose that amid the confusion of so many competing factors, the historical variability of ethical creeds may be more than random and perhaps I would not be the first writer to read an overall trajectory into the ethics of human relations.

This perceived trend commonly describes a progressive widening of the ethical 'net' which might be considered to run from some time long past when – it is assumed – only a favoured few such as the band or immediate family would benefit from any presumption of social consideration, through a gradual process of literate civilisation, with ever-larger settlements and wider political units offering greater security and trading opportunities but requiring the systematisation of respect for peers' interests. The modern norm, of course, says that all human beings should enjoy a range of basic human rights as enshrined in the *Universal Declaration of Human Rights.*

Imperfect though the concept's enactment may be, individual freedom has come to be presumed inalienable. Ownership of one person by another is fundamentally unacceptable. This is taken for granted. And, of course, it does not stop there: this process encompasses such developments as the decline of capital punishment, anti-racism, the emancipation of women and universal suffrage. In the West, at least, few dispute the desirability of these trends.

AND ANIMALS?

There have probably always been those who have argued for more humane treatment of all animals – Pythagoras and George Bernard Shaw being two of the more famous – either for the sake of the beast or for the good of our own bodies and souls. But however passionately propounded, until recently these tended to be voices in the western wilderness, whilst the rest of society got on with the serious business of harnessing other animals' bodies to economic advantage. Indeed, western civilisation is fairly literally built upon the bodies of other animals.

The Cartesian dogma that (being devoid of God-given souls) lesser species were mere insentient creatures is more fully observed today by industrially sponsored scientists, technologists and food producers than ever it was in the philosopher's lifetime. This crucially self-serving premise is routinely passed off as value-free scientific common sense while being used to pardon, for example, intensive animal production and genetic experimentation. The physical and behavioural modification which human technologies have imposed on creatures of other species could only have reached their current degree in a culture that denies the latter any element of personhood. Indeed, the parallels with discredited eugenic experimentation may yet come back to haunt an industry that has now proceeded far in advance of informed public consent.

It is unnecessary to take sides in the modern animal rights debate in order to perceive the arbitrary categorical distinction that denies non-humans protection from behaviour that is normally condemned out of hand if directed at other human beings. Not all is gloomy for advocates of animal liberation, however; the extension of ethical consideration beyond human beings has also advanced significantly in some spheres. It is a movement which has achieved some limited success in imposing legal constraints, at least locally, on the allowable impact by both industry and science upon many species' welfare. Particularly since the nineteenth century a duty of care for pets and farm animals has been enshrined in law, and even abstract entities such as habitats or wilderness zones are increasingly being accepted to have interests which deserve to be taken into account.

Meanwhile, just as the slaughter of living beings for sport or fashion has seen little short of a sea-change in its rapidly declining degree of public acceptability, so techniques regarding the breeding, raising, transport and slaughter of beasts have become the subject of increasing ethical debate within popular discourse. Even within recent decades, both moral positions and daily habits have altered appreciably. Some examples of these changes are listed below.

First, the number of people following a vegetarian diet has risen steadily for most of this century. The phenomenon of ethical or voluntary vegetarianism (as distinct from the traditional vegetarianism of large regions of the globe), along with its many variants such as 'demi-vegetarianism' (see Willetts, this volume) is now internationally established, but is furthest advanced in the US, the UK, Germany, Holland, Australia and some other 'developed' nations. While vegetarianism was once an occasional eccentricity, it is now prudent to verify guests' tastes in advance when catering for a dinner party or other gathering. Even veganism – the avoidance of all animal produce – today describes a significant part of the British population (around 1–2 per cent), whilst in sectors of the population such as female students a quarter or more say they are vegetarian or at least are refusing red meat.

Second, the marketing of meat is changing. The traditional butcher's shop selling flesh by the pound hewn from carcasses dripping blood is now deeply unfashionable, frequented largely by the middle-aged and elderly. The mode instead is either to promote meat ready-cooked in sesame buns whose char-browned 'patty', multiple dressings and crisp vegetable accompaniments ensure that most of the potentially distressing association with the beast is sublimated, or alternatively to retail the conceptually awkward substance in anonymously hygienic vacuum packs and pre-garnished ready meals in the reassuringly safe surroundings of supermarkets. Even the Director General of the British Meat and Livestock Commission no longer denies that this process serves to dissociate the product from the death of living animals, and thus reflects the consumer's desire not to be 'reminded of the animal from which the meat originated' (*Meat*, BBC2 TV, April 1995). Driven by the relentless but short-term pressures to maximise revenues for its clients, the industry is unwilling, unable, or quite probably conceptually ill-equipped to tackle this critical contemporary problem of its product's deeply ambivalent identity. Instead it has resorted to advertising's hardiest perennial by deploying a series of glossy but unsubtle images which seek to persuade us to buy more meat in order to enjoy sex more often (the 'food of love' campaign).

Third, meat's once unquestioned reputation as a vital component of any healthy diet has rapidly been losing its status. Not long ago, almost any doctor or nutritionist would confidently assert that eating plenty of protein was the key priority for every man, woman and child to grow healthy and strong. Distant peoples dependent upon less advantaged national economies were pitied for the protein gap they suffered as a result of their incapacity to subsist upon animal flesh as a staple of their cuisine. Now, the all-but-unanimous message from medicine and the media is to reduce meat consumption in favour of fresh fruit and vegetables, to achieve a balanced diet. Whether expressed in terms of fat-avoidance or fibre-deficit, meat is now the malign presence immanent in this discourse. This reversal in nutritional wisdom is normally explained as science having improved its understanding of the effect of too many saturated fats upon the incidence of heart disease. But science, true to form, may very well just be providing us with the rational reasoning required, whilst a more fundamental shift in the cultural climate occurs. After all, contented obesity used to be a sign of affluence and physical well-being, as it continues to be over large parts of the planet. Perhaps the deeper question is why long life appears to have been eclipsing quality of life as western society's apparent holy grail. A fuller answer may lie in the changing ecological and ideological environment as much as in improvements in medical knowledge, as I discuss below.

THE NEW RADICALISM

First, however, let us consider further the changing moral climate with regard to the use of other animals. For, as the middle ground has shifted, a new radicalism has emerged in the movement towards compassion. Examples of this new mood include the following.

First, the wearing of furs, almost overnight, has been transformed (in the UK at least) from an image of chic prestige to one of wanton selfishness. The decline and fall of this market in only a few years was precipitated chiefly by a highly effective awareness campaign by the now-bankrupted 'Lynx' (its name a deliberate pun) designed to highlight the links between the fashion and the death of animals. But whilst the anti-fur message was being brought to millions by expensive media campaigns, its central statement that killing for vanity was now socially unacceptable was crucially if controversially driven home by the activities of a few committed individuals armed with cans of spray paint.

Second, Greenpeace has developed from marginal extremism at its emergence to become one of the world's most famous and effective pressure groups. The organisation's campaigning was founded on the simple idea of direct action to protect endangered (and typically emotionally evocative) species such as dolphins and whales. Yet, even within this short period, the group has come to be perceived by many activists as having 'joined the establishment' by preferring talk to direct action. So in its wake follow yet more radical groups such as Sea Shepherd, who go so far as actually to sink illegal whaling vessels, Earth First!, Reclaim the Streets, and countless grassroots environmental groupings whose principal unifying feature is their refusal to be pigeon-holed as single-issue campaigns. These new ecological protest groups, in only a few years, have scored some significant successes in questioning, subverting and even changing official policies regarding road-building, land ownership, banking investments, and a host of other environmental and social issues. Through their 'DIY culture' they promote a throroughly distinct vision of the past and present as well as of a future which involves an expanding and increasingly self-reliant and self-referential subculture. In the emergent political manifesto of this new society of cultural dissent, respect for other animals is a crucial corollary of respect for other people and for the planet, and is revealed in the *de facto* norm of vegetarian if not vegan habits.

Third, the hunting of foxes, deer and game birds has become an increasingly beleaguered sport, disliked by a rising majority of the public, and actively opposed by a well-organised protest movement, despite political efforts to protect its participants' pleasures by criminalising the saboteurs. As I write, coincidentally on the 'glorious' twelfth of August when the British hunting season opens for the year, a television viewers' poll is published declaring 83 per cent of respondents to oppose grouse shooting (ITV Teletext, 12 Aug. 1996). Even fishing – often described as the nation's most popular participatory recreation – now finds itself subject to similar attentions. Any activity in which animals suffer purely for people's recreational pleasure is now likely to receive overwhelming disapproval from the public at large. Most local councils now ban circuses with animal acts from performing in their area, and any new movie release featuring animals now carries a routine declaration that they have been supervised by welfare officers, to pre-empt possible protest.

Fourth, protests over exports of live animals from the UK for slaughter abroad have been one manifestation at which even the middle aged and middle class turn out *en masse*, with large parts of the populations of port-towns declaring their shame at local facilities being the conduit for a trade that is seen as causing quite unnecessary levels of suffering. The campaigners advance arguments both about the stresses involved in the long-distance transportation of animals and about the production of veal in conditions long banned in the UK but still permitted overseas. Such debates have raged in small circles for many years, but now, as conditions have changed, the time has become right for wider exposure. A significant aspect of this argument has been the moral duty advanced for the UK not to permit animals reared here to be sent abroad to endure conditions no longer legal here – an extra-territorial extension of British sentiments which effectively claims some right of 'citizenship' and hence lifelong protection under UK law for beasts born within British borders. This cuts across basic principles of the system of free trade devised for corporate interests, which define non-humans, in effect, as goods on a par with any other raw material and for which the question of rights would never be considered even to arise. Thus, as in many other related contexts, the very presumptions on which the modern economic system operates are being questioned, sometimes very actively, by ordinary people. Despite a virtual news blackout as the media has moved on to new issues with new angles, the protests continue from one year to the next, as the trade carries on.

Finally, there has also been an upsurge in more extreme actions such as the firebombing of meat wholesalers and livestock transport firms, as well as the breaking of butchers' shop windows, much of which goes unreported. Punitive sentences indicate the perceived scale of threat to established interests, yet such illegal behaviour can and does achieve at least some of its aims. Major stores have largely ceased selling furs and, privately at least, admit that the unwelcome publicity as well as direct costs attendant upon criminally intimidatory tactics have been critical factors in their decisions. Similarly, both the increased security costs and the higher wages which vivisection laboratories complain of having to pay to attract sufficiently qualified staff in a field considered both unfashionable and potentially dangerous, must, by simple economics if for no other reason, diminish the scale of that branch of industry. It is politically unpopular to concede that 'terrorism' can succeed, though if it had no gains then it would surely be less common. But the long-term significance of such extremist activity is usually cited as evidence of deep-rooted despair at perceived injustices in a situation of obdurate immutability. The unique feature of this modern movement is that not only does it protest on behalf of others, but of other species. The circle of compassionate consideration is thus being widened by force.

THE FUTURE OF MEAT-EATING

In this context, then, my intention here is to consider whether meat's recent precipitous decline is indeed but a passing fad, or whether it is only the most recent development in a longer-term cultural trend. Will the day come when the idea of feeding on the flesh of other animals is universally abhorred, or even outlawed? Perhaps posterity will wonder what all the fuss was about, once some fresh philosophical consensus enables new regulations governing the humane rearing and shipment of livestock to achieve common consent. In other words, in fifty or a hundred years time, will this issue be a mere footnote in history or will normal standards have changed so much that future generations will regard current treatment of other animals with a horror similar to the modern view of slavery? Or, a third possibility, will a similar scale and style of protests (or even more) still be happening? This last possibility – of little change – seems the least likely of the three.

To gain some historical perspective on arguments which all too rarely are debated without either factional posturing or fraught polemicism, neither the statistics, nor even the rights and wrongs of the moral arguments, are sufficient. For the struggle to win hearts and minds is about far more than merely whether it is right to eat meat, or hunt foxes. These issues are suffused with layers of contemporary debate, which touch on much else besides the immediately apparent points at stake.

Indeed, animal concern has probably always been at least partly a metaphor for other social discourses. One example might be James Turner's (1980) suggestion that compassion is no 'natural instinct', but flourished in Victorian England as a sort of 'psychological bulwark against modernisation' because the world had changed so much and so rapidly that it became necessary. He suggests that it is no coincidence that the Royal Society for the Prevention of Cruelty to Animals (RSPCA), established in 1824, significantly pre-dates the National Society for the Protection of Children (NSPCC). It may further be noted that, of the two, only the animal charity enjoys royal accreditation.

A second example of how animal concern has always involved other issues could be Coral Lansbury's (1985) observation that, by and large, it was Victorian women who populated the early anti-vivisection movement. Lansbury suggests this was partly because this apparently non-mainstream social debate provided a covert but nonetheless subversive context for discussing the excesses of patriarchal gynaecology. Indeed it may be significant that it remains women who make up much of the memberships of animal rights groups to this day (in contrast to environmental organisations campaigning on issues in the 'public' sphere which tend to be male-dominated) – quite possibly as a continuing forum for disputing masculine hegemony.

However convincing these observations may be as partial explanations for some highly complex forms of social engagement, the prominence of animal issues in the contemporary consciousness cannot be accounted for adequately purely by reference to feminism, or even to human liberty. Beneath the modern animal exploitation debate lies another hugely unresolved but increasingly pressing issue which concerns the entire basis on which humanity *should* behave in relation not only to the rest of the human species, but also towards the natural world as a whole. This is a debate whose time has arrived because, in a very real sense, what is being discussed 'through' meat and other animal issues is essentially the cultural crisis of the late industrial era. There are at least two obvious ways in which this is occurring.

The first is the probably inevitable catharsis of a historical period which can only be close to having run its course. Though few are often conscious of it, many of the key ideological foundations on which modern western interpretations and judgements are based – particularly at the level of official discourse, such as in politics, commerce and in the mass media – were distilled amid the great western paradigm-shift led by figures like Descartes, Bacon and Hume as recently as the fifteenth to eighteenth centuries. These include the exaltation of principles such as abstract rationalism, physical reductionism, mind–body dualism and, above all, material determinism, all of which found some of their most significant symbolic expression through the treatment of the natural world. As Keith Thomas puts it, 'Man's dominion over nature was the self-consciously proclaimed ideal of early modern scientists' (1983: 29).

This cosmology denies non-human living beings any recognition of personhood, and was deployed to legitimise the wholesale exploration and colonisation of both the animate and inanimate worlds, and ultimately to excuse any treatment that might be convenient in pursuit of material and recreational desires. It is also a cosmology which has come effectively to divorce modern *homo urbanis* from many of the traditionally significant experiences and relationships with the ecosystem to an extent that most other periods in history would consider quite bizarre. This philosophy has paid huge material dividends, enabling a golden age of science and industry. However, an ideology appropriate to this peculiar period of rapid material expansionism perhaps makes less sense in a context where so many (amongst the better-off especially) are assessing the scale of concomitant social, spiritual and ecological losses, and proposing that more of the same is neither what is needed, nor wanted. We have recently learned to see science as 'simultaneously real, social and narrated' (Latour 1993: 7). A new scepticism amongst the body politic may not reject science wholesale, but does recognise that its self-serving and self-referential agendas and distorted representations belie its claims to objectivity, and have contributed to some of its (at least locally) catastrophic consequences (Gusterson 1996). In other words, the ideology of perpetual materialist growth may be approaching redundancy in part due to technology's success in meeting the population's material needs, and in part through its failures due to overestimating its own competence.

The second reason for the contemporary cultural crisis is related, but perhaps even more pressing. This is the looming spectre of global environmental catastrophe not only in terms of a senti-mental sense of loss, but as a highly rational fear for the species' very future expressed by the planet's leading scientific bodies, such as NASA, a succession of UN environment conferences, and even individualist politicians (e.g. Thatcher 1988); only the most optimistic technocrats (e.g. Baarschers 1996) or representatives of vested interests now deny that an effective collapse of global ecosystems is a real and present danger, albeit on an unknowable time-scale. No longer can it be assumed that today's children will enjoy even the same prosperity as now. Simple arithmetic – never mind Malthus – dictates that exponential growth in consumption of a finite planet's material funds cannot continue indefinitely. Moreover, the physical, political and, indeed, psycho-logical processes which apparently predicate that so many trends identified as threats (such as loss of biodiversity, or forest and fossil fuel conversion to CO_2) continue to worsen, rather than improve, seem inexorable. Suddenly, there is a sobering suspicion at large that survival, individually and as a species, cannot be taken for granted. This often erratic and nebulous anxiety inflects, for example, the surge in concern for health and fitness of recent years, as one part of the population, at least, reckons to counter these uncontrollable and often intangible threats through steps designed to maintain at least a comforting illusion of personal protection. By taking up exercise, stopping smoking, abstaining from alcohol or refusing red meat, some hope to maximise their own chances in a world of invisible dangers.

Few retain much faith in the traditional authorities' ability, or even intention, to look after us (Béjin 1976), and even fewer trust the experts to put things right. Many ancient certainties are up for grabs, and old institutions are newly open to challenge. Ulrich Beck (1992) calls this 'reflexive modernisation': a deep disenchantment with traditional forms of authority, including the family, unions, the Church, science in general, and all forms of industrial and political corporatism, in favour of an uncertainty that he ascribes to the transition from industrialism to a global 'risk' society.

As far as food is concerned, for example, surveys show that few believe 'they' *can* look after us, and fewer still that there is even any attempt to put the people's best interests first (see Keane, this volume). It is not only diehard cynics who accuse politicians of prioritising commercial profit above public interest. For example, it does little to build public confidence when it is revealed that more than three quarters (78 per cent) of the UK government's appointed 'independent' advisers on food and health receive money from multinational food and chemical firms whose primary interest – indeed, primary duty – is the maximisation of corporate profits (Hencke 1995).

Most major environmental issues have followed a characteristic pattern of initial official dismissal as 'fringe lunacy' only to be appropriated later by mainstream scientists and politicians who then continue to trivialise the public's role in crystallising the dangers (Grove-White 1993), failing to recognise the crucial role of myth and muddle in translating scientific facts into an agenda for necessary social action. So, similarly, each 'scare' about bugs or mad cows that shakes public confidence in the system which supplies foodstuffs, whose actual provenance is usually barely known, meets with official admonishments which insist there is absolutely no 'scientific' cause for concern (see Reilly and Miller, this volume). Yet by dismissing out of hand the population's rational reluctance to deliver blind trust, and by rubbishing popular construals of impenetrable scientific topics, such blandishments only precipitate yet stronger apprehensions that the substantial population of largely passive consumers is somehow being mis-fed, and misled. Thus, much as Hirschman (1970) describes, many people denied a voice in the discourse of science, of ecological concerns and of food scares, vote with their feet by abandoning the official constructs in order to establish their own alternatives. Too much has gone too far wrong for us to keep faith in the miracle cure-all just around the corner. That something needs to change is clear – and change so radical can occur only at the level of cultural values, rather than further technological fixes. Many of those not burying their heads in the sand, or wallowing in self-destructive nihilism and despair, are experimenting with new approaches, new belief systems (many of them in actuality very old), new commitments (including fundamentalist political and religious philosophies of many hues), and also the many so-called alternative lifestyles encompassing spiritual paths, complementary health systems, environmental pressure groups and behaviours such as meat avoidance.

Why meat avoidance? The reason is intractably bound up with meat's seminal importance as a symbol of the old order being challenged. The hegemonic ideology in recent centuries has been primarily about the extension of human power through scientific and technological prowess. Life itself has been industrialised in pursuit of maximising material affluence, and consumption of meat has been of central significance in demonstrating (western) humanity's quasi-divine mastery of the planet. It is, as I have argued elsewhere, this capacity to symbolise human domination of the material world which gives meat its prestige and 'macho' reputation for strength and virility (Fiddes 1991).

But today, the philosophy of conquering all seems to be bringing not safety but greater insecurity. Perhaps partly inspired by the prospect of the new millennium, the late twentieth century has seen all sorts of odd bedfellows – from the Churches to dissident economists, and from the popular media to some scholarly commentators – counsel that the time may be approaching when gratification and growth will need to be measured less in conspicuous displays of possession, and more in such qualities as physical and mental health, as well as social affirmation and spiritual enlightenment (e.g. Hancock 1986, Nordhaus and Tobin 1971, Dauncey 1988). As Mary Douglas puts it, we 'must talk threateningly about time, money, God and nature if we hope to get anything done. We must believe in the limitations and boundaries of nature which our community projects' (1975: 242, 245–6). This is, of course, not a new debate, but ecological urgency has given it new meaning. In 1943, Maslow observed that material needs are of a relatively low order in the hierarchy of human fulfilment, and that once such basic needs are met only the satisfaction of 'higher' needs such as belongingness, self-esteem and self-actualisation can meaningfully increase the quality of life. Such ideas have made little headway in permeating official thought. Certainly, politicians talk of regenerating a sense of community, or restoring people's feelings of self-worth, or renewing great moral debates, but all too often as if uttering ritual incantations, or in order to score a cheap political point.

Nonetheless, there are unmistakable signs of renewed public desire for greater integrity between personal beliefs and economic activity – and one of the most common manifestations of this is the notion of being sensitive to the ecological relationships in which everyone is unavoidably engaged in the course of daily behaviour. Demonstrating affinity with like-minded souls wherever they may be is part of that agenda. Refusing to eat the flesh of other animals is in many respects the ideal expression of rejecting the old technocratic world-view. As more people demand foods they can 'trust', the highly industrialised meat production machine has become a key avenue for rebellion. Few hope to master all the arcane economic, ecological or ethical arguments, but many nonetheless uphold their right to express their own perception of simple truths through one realm that remains within most people's own control – their daily consumption for sustenance. Thus, natural eating is almost synonymous with vegetarianism, perhaps not on the pages of the *Lancet* or the *Financial Times*, but certainly on *Neighbours*, which may in the end matter more.

In absolute numbers, vegetarianism remains a distinctly minority commitment. However, it continues to grow, as do numbers of people avoiding red meat or adopting veganism. Interestingly, however, meat sales have hardly fallen. The reason is that sales in some sectors of the market – particularly fast food – have also risen. These counterpoised trends suggest that tension between the two must surely rise, with some catharsis not far down the line.

It is possible, indeed likely, that as the debate crystallises and some positions become entrenched, more and increasingly radical anti-meat activities will continue to emerge, perhaps similar to the non-violent direct-action political theatre pioneered in recent years by anti-motorway and other environmental campaigners. As this occurs, if it does, it seems certain that government and industry, apparently still entrenched in their seventeenth-century ideology of mechanistic materialism, will struggle to respond to a public mood that it cannot understand let alone incorporate. But its complaints about people's 'sentimentality' and 'lack of realism' will only stoke up the fires of discontent, propelling us more rapidly towards a revolution in what is accepted as everyday 'common sense'.

CONCLUSION

All the foregoing might be taken to suggest that meat is inexorably on the way out. This is by no means the case. Certainly it is possible – for all the reasons outlined above – but it is not inevitable. There have been many (generally small-scale) societies which have combined a culture of respect or indeed reverence towards nature in general, and animals in particular, with a way of life which includes killing and eating them. Arguably, an ideal ecological society would practise integrated organic farming, mixing livestock with crops, in which not to use the flesh of redundant animals at least would be wasteful (see Willetts, this volume). This has been the pattern for most of history, after all, and there is little reason why it should not be so again in the future.

Even today, the issue for many who declare a problem with consuming the products of the modern meat industry is not a simple matter of whether or not to kill, but concerns the manner in which other animals are treated in the process of producing the flesh for food. Many 'ethical vegetarians', often reverting from total vegetarianism, will eat meat from beasts they believe to have been reared in conditions they consider acceptable, but refuse the products of industrial agriculture. In theory, at least, it is not beyond possibility that western society's mood might migrate in this direction, rather than towards a total taboo on meat-eating.

However, the interests which continue to propel the state towards excluding moral and indeed emotional considerations from matters it deems the exclusive preserve of profitability have formidable momentum, and maintain a powerful grip on the levers of authority. A recent example is genetic manipulation, which has brought about, with scant public debate or even awareness, the public sale of various novel foods.

If a free market in the genetics of living organisms is tolerated, in defiance of the tide of public feeling, then meat may yet become the symbolic centrepiece of a cultural revolution on a scale unprecedented since the Enlightenment. That conceptual catharsis marked the passing of God's omnipotence. This one would mark the passing of our own, by further spreading the net of moral inclusivity defining what – one might even say *whom* – may be treated as mere property, to be disposed of in whatever manner makes someone a profit, and what has rights.

REFERENCES

Baarschers, W. (1996) *Eco-facts and Eco-fiction*, London: Routledge.
Beck, U. (1992) *Risk Society: Towards a New Modernity*, London: Sage.

Béjin, A. (1976) 'Crise des valeurs, crise des mesures', *Communications* 25: 39–72.

Dauncey, G. (1988) *After the Crash*, Basingstoke, Hants: Green Print.

Douglas, M. (1975) *Implicit Meanings*, London: Routledge and Kegan Paul.

Fiddes, N. (1991) *Meat: A Natural Symbol*, London: Routledge.

Grove-White, R. (1993) 'Environmentalism: a new moral discourse for technological society?', in K. Milton (ed.) *Environmentalism: The View from Anthropology*, London: Routledge.

Gusterson, H. (1996) 'Nuclear weapons testing: scientific experiment as political ritual', in Laura Nader (ed.) *Naked Science*, London: Routledge.

Hancock, T. (1986) 'Health-based indicators of economic progress', in Paul Ekins (ed.) *The Living Economy*, London: Routledge and Kegan Paul.

Hencke, D. (1995) 'Labour attacks health quangos on advisers' links with firms', *Guardian* 14 July: 5.

Hirschman, A.O. (1970) *Exit, Voice and Loyalty: Responses to Decline in Firms, Organizations and States*, Cambridge, MA: Harvard University Press.

Lansbury, C. (1985) 'Gynaecology, pornography, and the anti-vivisection movement', *Victorian Studies* 28: 413–37.

Latour, B. (1993) *We Have Never Been Modern*, London: Harvester Wheatsheaf.

Maslow, A.H. (1943) 'A theory of human motivation', *Psychological Review* 50: 370–96.

Nordhaus, W.D. and Tobin, J. (1971) 'Is growth obsolete?', in M. Moss (ed.) *The Measurement of Economic and Social Performance*, Princeton: Princeton University Press.

Thatcher, M. (1988) *Speech to the Royal Society*, London: Conservative Party.

Thomas, K. (1983) *Man and the Natural World*, Harmondsworth: Penguin.

Turner, J. (1980) *Reckoning with the Beast: Animals, Pain, and Humanity in the Victorian Mind*, Baltimore: Johns Hopkins University Press.

Index